Biology of the Neonate

Foetal and Neonatal Research

Founded 1959 as 'Biologia Neonatorum' by A. Minkowski
(formerly 'Etudes Néo-Natales')

KARGER

Printed in Switzerland
on acid-free paper by
Thür AG Offsetdruck, Pratteln

Appears monthly:
2 volumes per year (12 issues)

Biology of the Neonate

Submission: Only original papers written in English are considered and should be sent to:

S. Karger AG
Editorial Dept. 'Biology of the Neonate'
P.O. Box
CH–4009 Basel (Switzerland)

Manuscripts should be submitted in triplicate (with three sets of illustrations of which one is an original), typewritten double-spaced on one side of the paper, with a wide margin.

Conditions: All manuscripts are subject to editorial review. Manuscripts are received with the explicit understanding that they are not under simultaneous consideration by any other publication. Submission of an article for publication implies the transfer of the copyright from the author to the publisher upon acceptance. Accepted papers become the permanent property of 'Biology of the Neonate' and may not be reproduced by any means, in whole or in part, without the written consent of the publisher. It is the author's responsibility to obtain permission to reproduce illustrations, tables, etc. from other publications.

Brief communications: Short reports, including case reports, brief laboratory observations, and preliminary communications, may be submitted for accelerated publication under 'brief communications'. To qualify for rapid publication, such reports should not exceed a printed length of two pages, i.e., generally not more than 1,000 words of text accompanied by 2 figures or tables and from 5 to 10 references.

Arrangement

Title page: The first page of each paper should indicate the title (main title underlined), the authors' names, and the institute where the work was conducted. A short title for use as running head as well as the full address of the author to whom correspondence should be sent are also required.

Key words: For indexing purposes, a list of 3–10 key words in English is essential.

Abstract: Each paper needs an abstract of up to 10 lines.

Small type: Paragraphs which can or must be set in smaller type (case histories, test methods, etc.) should be indicated with a 'p' (petit) in the margin on the left-hand side.

Footnotes: Avoid footnotes. When essential, they are numbered consecutively and typed at the foot of the appropriate page.

Tables and illustrations: Tables and illustrations (both numbered in Arabic numerals) should be prepared on separate sheets. Tables require a heading and figures a legend, also prepared on a separate sheet. For the reproduction of illustrations, only good drawings and original photographs can be accepted; negatives or photocopies cannot be used. When possible, group several illustrations on one block for reproduction (max. size 144 × 196 mm) or provide crop marks. On the back of each illustration, indicate its number, the author's name, and 'top'. Color illustrations are reproduced at the author's expense.

References: In the text identify references by Arabic numerals [in square brackets]. Material submitted for publication but not yet accepted should be noted as 'unpublished data' and not be included in the reference list. The list of references should include only those publications which are cited in the text. Do not alphabetize; number references in the order in which they are first mentioned in the text. The surnames of the authors followed by initials should be given. There should be no punctuation other than a comma to separate the authors. Cite all authors, 'et al' is not sufficient. Abbreviate journal names according to the Index Medicus system. (Also see International Committee of Medical Journal Editors: Uniform requirements for manuscripts submitted to biomedical journals. Br Med J 1988;296:401–405.)

Examples

(a) Papers published in periodicals: Kauffman HF, van der Heide S, Beaumont F, Blok H, de Vries K: Class-specific antibody determination against *Aspergillus fumigatus* by means of the enzyme-linked immunosorbent assay. III. Comparative study: IgG, IgA, IgM ELISA titers, precipitating antibodies and IgE binding after fractionation of the antigen. Int Arch Allergy Appl Immunol 1986;80:300–306.

(b) Monographs: Matthews DE, Farewell VT: Using and Understanding Medical Statistics. Basel, Karger, 1985.

(c) Edited books: Hardy WD Jr, Essex M: FeLV-induced feline acquired immune deficiency syndrome: A model for human AIDS; in Klein E (ed): Acquired Immunodeficiency Syndrome. Prog Allergy. Basel, Karger, 1986, vol 37, pp 353–376.

Full address: The exact postal address complete with postal code must be given at the bottom of the title page. Please supply also Phone and Fax numbers.

Further details: Authors may consult our leaflet 'Rules for the Preparation of Manuscripts', available on request from the Publisher, S. Karger AG, P.O. Box, CH–4009 Basel (Switzerland).

Page charges: There is no page charge for papers of 6 or fewer printed pages (including tables, illustrations and references). Each additional complete or partial page is charged to the author at SFr. 225.– / US $ 150.00. The allotted size of a paper is equal to approx. 12 manuscript pages (including tables, illustrations and references).

Galley proofs: Unless indicated otherwise, galley proofs are sent to the first-named author and should be returned with the least possible delay. Alterations made in galley proofs, other than the correction of printer's errors, are charged to the author. No page proofs are supplied.

Reprints: Order forms and a price list are sent with the galley proofs. Orders submitted after the issue is printed are subject to considerably higher prices. Allow five weeks from date of publication for delivery of reprints.

KARGER

General Information

Biology of the Neonate

Publication data: 'Biology of the Neonate' is published 12 times annually. Volumes 65–66 with 6 issues each appear in 1994.

Subscription rates: Subscriptions run for a full calendar year. Prices are given per volume.

Personal subscription:

Subscription + postage and handling
SFr. 319.90 + SFr. 15.60 Europe
SFr. 319.90 + SFr. 23.40 Overseas
US$ 213.50 + US$ 15.60
(Must be in the name of, billed to, and paid by an individual. Order must be marked 'personal subscription'.)

Institutional subscription:

Subscription + postage and handling
SFr. 457.– + SFr. 24.– Europe
SFr. 457.– + SFr. 36.– Overseas
US$ 305.00 + US$ 24.00

Airmail postage: SFr. 36.–, US$ 30.00. (Extra per volume.)

Discount subscription prices:
Neonatal Society;
Société Française de Néonatologie.

Microform edition: SFr. 288.50, US$ 152.50. (Available exclusively to subscribers of the paper edition.)

Subscription orders: Orders can be placed at agencies, bookstores, directly with the Publisher S. Karger AG, P.O. Box, CH – 4009 Basel (Switzerland)
or with any of the following distributors:

Deutschland: S. Karger GmbH, Postfach
D – 79095 Freiburg

France: Librairie Luginbühl
36, bd de Latour-Maubourg
F-75007 Paris

Great Britain, Ireland: S. Karger Publishers
11 Ravenscroft Road
Beckenham, Kent BR3 4TP

USA: S. Karger Publishers, Inc.
26 West Avon Road, P.O. Box 529
Farmington, CT 06085

India, Bangladesh, Sri Lanka:
S. Karger India Subscription Agency
B – 5/132 Safdarjung Enclave
New Delhi-110029

Japan: Katakura Libri, Inc.
36-9 Hongo 3-chome, Bunkyo-ku
Tokyo 113

Change of address: Both old and new address should be sent to the subscription source.

Single issues and back volumes: Information can be obtained through the Publisher.

Advertising: Correspondence and rate requests should be addressed to the Publisher.

Bibliographic indices: This journal is regularly listed in bibliographic services, including *Current Contents®*.

Book Reviews: Books are accepted for review by special agreement.

Guidelines for Disk Submission

Karger Publishers welcomes the submission of manuscripts on disk.

Please observe the 'Instructions to authors' as well as the following guidelines:

Technical Data

The preferred **storage medium** is a 3.5- or 5.25-inch disk in MS-DOS format. Macintosh is also acceptable.

The preferred **word processing package** is Microsoft Word. Other commonly used PC text programs are also accepted, as well as ASCII formats.

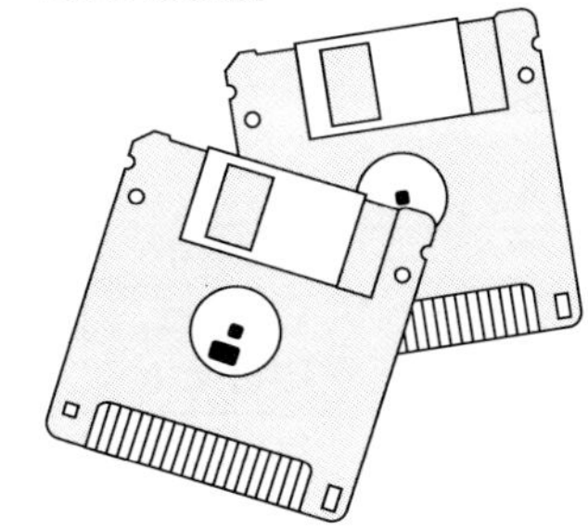

Handling

All manuscripts accepted for Karger publications are subject to copyediting. It is therefore essential that you send us a **double-spaced printout** of your manuscript which exactly matches the disk.

Any subsequent revised versions should be clearly marked as such, both on the disk and on the manuscript.

The copyedited manuscript and the disk will be returned to you along with the galley proofs. Please be sure to **check the galleys against the manuscript** in which changes introduced by the copyeditor and/or questions will be marked.

Please **label** your disk with (a) the title of the journal for which it is submitted, (b) a short version of the paper title, (c) your name and (d) the software and hardware used.

Text Arrangement

Text and headings should be ranged left throughout, without word breaks. **Do not center, space, or use block letters** for text and headings (except for abbreviations). **Do not use indentations** to mark the beginning of a paragraph, but use one blank line between paragraphs.

Be sure to use the **same type style for headings of the same ranking** throughout the text.

When using **special characters** not available on a standard keyboard (including Greek characters), please do so by a readily identifiable code, and use the same code throughout the manuscript. Supply a **complete list of the codes used** at the beginning of the text.

Illustrations, tables and mathematical formulae will be handled conventionally.

KARGER

Control of Breathing during Development

Apnea of the Newborn and in Sudden Infant Death Syndrome

Colloquium
Nancy-Pont-à-Mousson,
France
September 7–9, 1992

Paul Vert, Nancy
Jacob V. Aranda, Montreal
Charlotte Catz, Bethesda, Md.
Sumner Yaffe, Bethesda, Md.

38 figures and 11 tables, 1994

KARGER

Scientific Committee

Chairperson
Prof. Maria Delivoria-Papadopoulos, Philadelphia

Prof. Jacob V. Aranda, Montreal
Prof. Sukhamay Lahiri, Philadelphia
Prof. Sumner Yaffe, Bethesda
Dr. Charlotte Catz, Bethesda
Prof. Claude Gaultier, Paris
Dr. Daniel Jordan, Lyon
Prof. Nicolas Kopp, Lyon
Prof. François Marchal, Nancy
Prof. Pierre Monin, Nancy
Prof. Paul Vert, Nancy

Local Organizing Committee

Paul Vert
Pierre Monin
Daniel Jordan
Nicolas Kopp
François Marchal
Jean-Pierre Crance
Marie-Jeanne Boutroy
Yves Badonnel
Astrid Nehlig
Aida Bairam
Jean-Michel Hascoet

Acknowledgments

The organization of this Colloquium and this publication has been made possible thanks to the financial support of the following organizations:

Institut National de la Santé et de la Recherche Médicale (INSERM);
National Institute of Child Health and Human Development (NIH);
Université de Nancy I – Faculté de Médecine;
District Urbain de l'Agglomération Nancéienne;
Conseil Général de Meurthe-et-Moselle;
Association Naître et Vivre;
Association pour la Recherche en Biologie et Médecine du Développement Humain.

We would like to thank the Drug and Nutrition Companies, particularly for their outstanding support:
Wellcome, Guigoz;

and for their great help:
Gallia, Kontron, Mead Johnson, Milupa, Serono, Nestlé, Crinex, Jacquemaire, Materna, Nutricia, Sodilac, Vickers.

S. Karger
Medical and Scientific Publishers
Basel · Freiburg · Paris · London
New York · New Delhi · Bangkok
Singapore · Tokyo · Sydney

Drug Dosage
The authors and the publisher have exerted every effort to ensure that drug selection and dosage set forth in this text are in accord with current recommendations and practice at the time of publication. However, in view of ongoing research, changes in government regulations, and the constant flow of information relating to drug therapy and drug reactions, the reader is urged to check the package insert for each drug for any change in indications and dosage and for added warnings and precautions. This is particularly important when the recommended agent is a new and/or infrequently employed drug.

Printed in Switzerland on acid-free paper by Thür AG Offsetdruck, Pratteln
ISBN 3-8055-5975-5

Contents

Biol Neonate 1994;65:133

Guest Editors
Paul Vert
Jacob V. Aranda
Charlotte Catz
Sumner Yaffe

Nancy/Montrcal/Bethesda, Md.

Foreword

Breathing control is one of the most vulnerable systems during development. Its disturbance accounts for a large amount of brain damage in the premature newborn and is a part of the complex mechanism which can lead to sudden infant death (SIDS). Although extensive information exists in the literature, the regulatory processes of breathing and their adaptation from fetal life to complete maturity remain poorly understood.

Thanks to Jean-Pierre Relier, Editor-in-Chief, this double issue of *Biology of the Neonate* assembles papers presented at a research colloquium on 'Control of Breathing during Development. Apnea of the Newborn and in Sudden Infant Death Syndrome' held in Nancy-Pont-à-Mousson, September 7–9, 1992. This meeting co-sponsored by l'Institut National de la Santé et de la Recherche Médicale (France) and The National Institute for Child Health and Human Development (NIH – USA) gathered pediatricians and fundamentalists from different fields of neurosciences and physiology coming from 12 European and North-American countries. During this meeting, a special Workshop was devoted to the neuropathological findings in SIDS victims in an attempt to reach a consensus on common procedures.

The vulnerability of the control of breathing in the neonatal period is best illustrated by the depressive effect of hypoxia on the respiratory drive. The most life-threatening phenomenon both in premature newborns and in infants at risk of sudden death is the delay or the absence of apnea offset.

If some approaches constitute exciting research tools such as medullary fetal cells inherently sensitive to CO_2 and pH changes, or the effects of repeated episodes of asphyxia on brain energy metabolism, the absence of experimental models remains a major handicap for the understanding of the pathophysiology of apnea.

The mystery of the chemosensory regulation of breathing and of its resetting at birth may begin to be understood thanks to advances in the physiology of neuromodulators like adenosine, dopamine, norepinephrine or serotonin and of the development of their receptors either peripherally or in the brain stem. This resetting may also explain the good luck of premature infants who have the benefit of changing from intermittent periods of fetal breathing to an almost regular respiratory drive at birth.

Since more and more very-low-birthweight infants are able to survive, apnea of prematurity becomes one of the main concerns in neonatal units. The recording of respiratory patterns with increasingly sophisticated monitors leads not only to the recognition of the true incidence of apnea but also to the characterization of different types related or not to sleep states, heart rate, obstruction, gastroesophageal reflux, etc. Transplacentally acquired depressants or beta-blockers may also induce apnea; however, their recognition and prevention are not always obvious.

If the pharmacological treatment of apnea, mainly with methylxanthines or doxapram, is widely prescribed, it remains symptomatic and somewhat empirical. The experimental data provided assess the efficacy of the respiratory stimulants only by measuring the ventilatory function. If the side effects of these drugs can be demonstrated in animal models, their effectiveness in preventing apnea has to be shown in the premature newborn itself.

We thank all the authors for their outstanding contributions during the meeting and in this publication. We hope they will not only provide comprehensive help for those who are faced with the clinical challenges but also promote scientific exchange.

Biol Neonate 1994;65:134–139

S. Lahiri

Department of Physiology, University of Pennsylvania School of Medicine, Philadelphia, Pa., USA

Carotid Body Chemoreception: Mechanisms and Dynamic Protection against Apnea

Key Words
Peripheral chemoreceptors
Central chemoreceptors
Carbonic anhydrase
Ion exchangers
Ion channels
Neurotransmitters
Dopamine
Oxidative metabolism
Heme pigments
Intracellular pH
Newborn

Abstract
A critical role of peripheral chemoreceptors in terminating apnea and in initiating normal breathing has been emphasized. Since these are the only organs which signal hypoxia, failure of its adequate development can contribute to the disease of respiratory failure in neonatal life. The failure may reside in any of the steps from initiation of O_2 chemoreception involving respiratory and non-respiratory pigments, ion balance including H^+ and Ca^{2+}, neurotransmitter mechanisms and transduction.

Apnea results in continuing depletion of systemic and cellular O_2 and accumulation of CO_2. Both O_2 depletion and CO_2 accumulation stimulate peripheral chemoreceptors whereas O_2 depletion exerts a depressant effect on the neural phrenic output and pulmonary ventilation, despite the stimulatory effects of CO_2 through mechanisms in the central nervous system. The neural output particularly from the carotid body initiates chemoreflexes controlling respiration and other autonomic neural functions [1]. The effects of hypoxia on the neurons in the central nervous system is complex but the resultant effect is a depression of the phrenic neural output and pulmonary ventilation [2, 3]. A good deal of the effects of hypoxia concerns ion balance of the neurons [4, 5]. Thus, two competing and antagonistic effects of hypoxia determine pulmonary ventilation and apnea. In the absence of peripheral chemoreceptor drive, the central depressant effect would dominate with life-threatening situation, for example in sudden infant death syndrome [6]. The focus of this paper is on the role of carotid body chemoreceptor function and its dynamic effects in the initiation and termination of apnea. The present model of carotid body function is that upon initiation of O_2 chemoreception by metabolic and membrane mechanisms involving heme pigments in the glomus cells, the intracellular Ca^{2+} is mobilized which assists neurotransmitter release and eventually chemosensory discharge.

Dr. S. Lahiri
Department of Physiology
University of Pennsylvania School of Medicine
Philadelphia, PA 19104-6085 (USA)

0006–3126/94/
0654–0134$5.00/0

Dependence of Apneic Threshold on Peripheral and Central Chemoreceptor Functions

The first point to establish is the importance of the peripheral chemoreceptor drive in initiating and terminating apnea. CO_2 plays critical roles in both carotid and central chemoreceptor functions. A sufficiently low P_{CO_2} can diminish carotid chemosensory activity near zero activity, and a sufficiently low central P_{CO_2} would eliminate chemoreflex effect of the chemosensory discharge [7]. The strength of hypoxia needed to elicit a response is greater at lower Pa_{CO_2}, both for carotid chemosensory activity and for ventilation. That is, the chemosensory input needed to break apnea is greater at lower Pa_{CO_2}. In the absence of the sensory input, Pa_{CO_2} needed to elicit ventilatory response is greater. During hypoxia, however, the central P_{O_2} would fall far, produce a depressant effect, and rhythmic ventilation would never start after a few abortive attempts.

The peripheral chemoreceptor drive, at a heightened gain, can also initiate apnea as seen in the periodic breathing at high altitude [8]. In this instance, the effect is accentuated by hypocapnia resulting from the increased peripheral drive and from a depressed central state during quiet sleep [9].

Cl^-/HCO_3^- Exchanger and O_2 Chemoreception

There are several ways that the exchanger function of the chemoreceptor glomus cells can be blocked. Zero or low HCO_3^- or Cl^- in the external medium, and pharmacological agents like DIDS and SITS can perform this function. We showed that absence of HCO_3^- in the external medium of an in vitro carotid body preparation significantly delayed and attenuated the chemosensory response to hypoxia. This effect is likely to be due to intracellular alkalosis [10]. DIDS and SITS exert additional effects. Thus, any defect in the Cl^--HCO_3^- ion exchange mechanisms would influence the chemosensory responses.

Carbonic Anhydrase and O_2 Chemoreception

Demonstration of the effect of carbonic anhydrase (CA) inhibition in the carotid body needs an in vitro carotid body preparation in order to avoid contribution of carbonic anhydrase in red blood cells which distorts the stimulus response relationship due to disequilibrium in the CO_2 hydration reaction in the circulating blood. Blockade of carbonic anhydrase with methazolamide (20 μM) which eliminated the fast response to CO_2 also delayed the response to hypoxia, although the maximal response was not significantly attenuated [11]. Thus, any deficiency of CA in the carotid body would influence the dynamic responses.

Ion Channels and O_2 Chemoreception

It has been reported that in the glomus cell membrane there is a special K^+ channel which is O_2 sensitive [12, 13]. However, its role in the physiological responses is not clear because its O_2 sensitivity lies in the high range of P_{O_2}, 150–80 Torr [12], unlike the chemosensory responses: arterial P_{O_2} <80 Torr, microvascular P_{O_2} <50 Torr and cell P_{O_2} <40 Torr [14].

Voltage-gated Ca^{2+} channel has been implicated [15, 16] for Ca^{2+} entry into glomus cell but has not been proven [17]. Effect of hypoxia is not perceptible on Ca^{2+} conductance in the glomus cell membrane [12], and

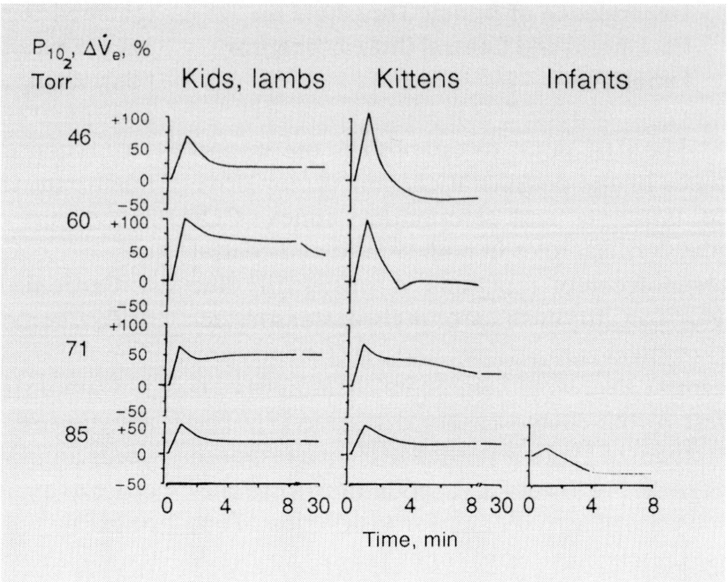

Fig. 1. Ventilatory responses to hypoxia at sea level. Comparison of the effects of low inspired P_{O_2} on ventilatory changes ($\triangle\dot{V}$%) in newborn kids and lambs (left-hand panel), kittens (middle panel) and human infants less than 72 h old. The ventilatory responses are normalized with respect to the resting ventilation in each species.

hypoxia may or may not increase intracellular $[Ca^{2+}]$ [15, 17, 18]. The $Ca^{2+}{}_i$ response may be independent of external $[Ca^{2+}]$ in the short run but dependent in the long run. The relative role of intra- and extracellular Ca^{2+} is not clear but its mobilization seems to be a part of the chemoreception process.

Neurotransmitter

There are both inhibitory and excitatory putative neurotransmitters in the glomus cells [19]. The dominant inhibitory one seems to be dopamine, and excitatory ones are substance P and acetylcholine. Dopamine exerts both inhibitory and excitatory effects in the newborn kittens but blockade of D_2 receptors invariably excites the chemoreceptors [20]. It is not clear what combination of these neurotransmitter-like agents determine the chemosensory response to hypoxia. Development of receptors for these agents is not known.

Chronic Hypoxia in the Newborn

Newborns at high altitudes are chronically hypoxic. Yet their ventilation is not significantly stimulated by moderate hypoxia [21]. Withdrawal of ambient hypoxia is not followed by any significant decrease in ventilation. Also, an additional brief period of hypoxia did not stimulate ventilation. Taken together, we concluded that hypoxic chemoreception was not adequately developed at high altitude. This is reminiscent of newborns' characteristics at sea level [22]. Continued hypoxia seems to delay development of hypoxic chemoreflex [22] particularly as seen in the young subjects with cyanotic congenital heart disease [23].

It is important to note that carotid body also respond to chronic hypoxia by cellular hypertrophy and hyperplasia and by increased concentrations and turnover rates of catecholamines [24]. This vigorous cellular response is not matched by the physiological response which is only rather mild.

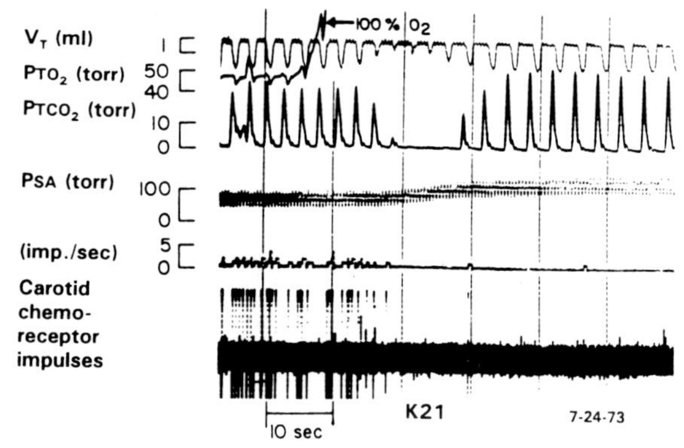

Fig. 2. Carotid chemoreceptor and chemoreflex responses in a 4-day-old kitten. Effects of transition from hypoxia to hyperoxia on carotid chemosensory discharge, ventilation and arterial blood pressure. Tracings from the top are tidal volumes (V_T), tracheal P_{O_2} (P_{TO_2}), tracheal P_{CO_2} (P_{TCO_2}), systemic arterial pressure (P_{SA}), carotid chemoafferent impulses per second and impulses.

Carotid Chemoreceptor and Ventilatory Chemoreflex in Newborns at Sea Level

In search of a model mimicking human responses, we measured ventilatory responses to hypoxic in several animal species. Figure 1 compares these responses with those of human newborns (taken from the literature). Alveolar P_{CO_2} was not maintained in these studies. In all the instances the fast peak was followed by less of a response. Newborn lambs and kids showed significant and sustained responses whereas kittens showed diminished sustained response as the intensity of hypoxic stimulus increased. Human newborns showed the least excitatory response.

An example of the simultaneously measured carotid chemosensory and ventilatory responses is shown in figure 2. During steady state hypoxia, a weak chemosensory response was seen. Raising inspired P_{O_2} promptly eliminated the chemosensory activity and transiently diminished tidal volumes. The chemoreceptor activity during hypoxia was far less than those in the cat carotid body [1, 20, 22]. The time-course of effects of oxygen on tidal volume and breath frequency was not fully correlated with the chemosensory activities. The effects of the state of oxygenation on brain and blood pressure are dissociated from those on the carotid chemoreceptors. The respiratory effects of hypoxia through the neuronal controller have been well demonstrated [2–5].

Metabolism and Membrane in O_2 Chemoreception

It has amply been demonstrated that metabolic inhibitors momentarily stimulate and then block O_2 chemoreception without attenuating the response to CO_2 and nicotine [25]. Blockade of oxidative metabolism of glomus cell also inhibited its hypoxic responses [17] due to blockade of intracellular Ca^{2+} release. There is, however, an alternative proposal that hypoxia decreases K^+ conductance and depolarizes the glomus cell [12, 13], allowing Ca^{2+} entry and neurotransmitter release. There is, however, a great deal of controversy on this issue at this point in time.

The issue of metabolic vs. membrane contribution to O_2 chemoreception can be tested with CO which competes with O_2. Cytochrome c oxidase is specifically inhibited by CO at high P_{CO} [26]. Using P_{CO} of 50–550 Torr at P_{O_2} levels of 50–150 Torr, we were able to show that CO blocked hypoxic effects through one mechanism and excited the chemosensory discharge through cytochrome c oxidase mechanism [unpubl. observations]. The latter was strongly inhibited by light. The conclusion is that the usual cytochrome oxidase and other heme pigment(s) participate in O_2 chemoreception in the carotid body. Accordingly, development and maintenance of these pigments are critical for O_2 chemoreception in the carotid body.

Failure of Peripheral Chemosensory Function

The peripheral chemoreceptors and the chemosensory function may fail under the hypoxic stress. We have observed the phenomenon in single [27] as well as in the whole carotid sinus nerves [unpubl. observations]. Wiemer and colleagues [28] described the phenomenon more completely. Clearly, oxidative energy is needed to support the chemosensory discharge, and there is a potential for its failure in prolonged apnea, making its termination impossible.

In summary, evidence has been presented to show that carotid body function is indispensable for the protection against the central depressant effect of hypoxia on pulmonary ventilation and is essential for normal termination of apnea. Accordingly, development of the factors which are responsible for the initiation and control of O_2 chemoreception and chemosensory response are critical issues during development.

Acknowledgement

I am grateful to Wendy Patriquin for her secretarial assistance. Supported in part by grant HL-43413.

References

1 Lahiri S: Peripheral chemoreflexes; in Crystall RG, West JB, Barnes PJ, Cherniack NS, Weibel ER (eds): The Lung. New York, Raven Press, 1991, pp 1333–1340.
2 Lahiri S: Depressant effect of acute and chronic hypoxia on ventilation; in Paintal AS (ed): Morphology and Mechanisms of Chemoreceptors. Delhi, University of Delhi, 1976, pp 138–145.
3 Richter DW: Responses of the medullary respiratory network of the cat to hypoxia. J Physiol (Lond) 1991;443:231–256.
4 Trippenbach T: Ionic environment in the central nervous system and effects of hypoxia in early life; in Haddad GG, Farber JP (eds): Developmental Neurobiology of Breathing. New York, Marcel Dekker, 1991, pp 643–660.
5 Jiang C, Xia Y, Caddad GC: Role of ATP-sensitive K^+ channels during anoxia: major differences between rat (newborn and adult) and turtle neurons. J Physiol 1992;448:599–612.
6 Pervin DG, Cutz E, Becker LE, Bryan AC, Madapallimatum A, Sole MJ: Sudden infant death syndrome: Increased carotid body dopamine and noradrenaline content. Lancet 1984;ii:535–537.
7 Lahiri S, Mokashi A, DeLaney RF, Fishman AP: Arterial P_{O_2} and P_{CO_2} stimulus threshold for carotid chemoreceptors and breathing. Respir Physiol 1978;34:359–375.
8 Lahiri S, Maret K, Sherpa MG: Dependence of high altitude sleep apnea in ventilatory sensitivity to hypoxia. Respir Physiol 1983;52:281–301.
9 Data AK, Shea SA, Horner RL, Guz A: The influence of induced hypocapnia and sleep on the endogenous respiratory rhythms in humans. J Physiol (Lond) 1991;440:17–33.
10 Iturriaga R, Lahiri S: Carotid body chemoreception in the absence and presence of CO_2-HCO_3^-. Brain Res 1991;568:253–260.
11 Iturriaga R, Lahiri S, Mokashi A: Carbonic anhydrase and chemoreception in the cat carotid body. Am J Physiol 1991;261:C565–573.
12 Lopez-Barneo J, Lopez-Lopez JR, Urena J, Gonzalez C: Chemotransduction in the carotid body: K^+ current modulated by PO_2 in type I chemoreceptor cells. Science 1988;241:580–582.
13 Delpiano MA, Heschler J: Evidence for a PO_2 sensitive K^+ channel in the type I cell of the rabbit carotid body. FEBS Lett 1989;249:195–198.

14 Lahiri S, Rumsey WL, Wilson DF, Iturriaga R: Control of microvascular PO_2 and chemoreception in the cat carotid body. J Appl Physiol 1993;in press.
15 Sato M, Ikada K, Yoshizaki K, Koyano H: Response of cytosolic calcium to anoxia and cyanide in cultured glomus cells of newborn rabbit carotid body. Brain Res 1991; 551:527–530.
16 Shirihata M, Fitzgerald RS: Dependence of hypoxic chemotransduction in cat carotid body on voltage-gated calcium channels. J Appl Physiol 1991;71:1062–1069.
17 Duchen MR, Biscoe TJ: Relative mitochondrial membrane potential and $[Ca^{2+}]_i$ in type I cells isolated from the rabbit carotid body. J Physiol (Lond) 1992;450:33–61.
18 Donnelley DF, Kholwadwala K: Hpyoxia decreases intracellular calcium in adult rat carotid body glomus cells. J Neurophysiol 1992;67: 1543–1551.
19 Fidone SJ, Gonzalez C, Dinger B, Gomez-Niño A, Obeso A, Yoshizaki K: Cellular aspects of peripheral chemoreceptor function; in Crystal RG, West JB, Barnes PJ, Cherniack NS, Weibel ER (eds): The lung. New York, Raven Press, 1991; pp 1319–1332.
20 Marchal F, Bairam A, Haonzi P, Hascoct JM, Crance JP, Vert P, Lahiri S: Dual responses of carotid chemosensory afferents in the newborn kitten. Respir Physiol 1992;87:183–193.
21 Lahiri S, Brody JS, Velasquez T, Motoyama EK, Simpser M, DeLaney RG, Polgar G: Pulmonary adaptation to high altitude: Genetic vs. environment. Nature 1976;261: 133–135.
22 Lagercrantz H, Milerad J, Walker D: Control of ventilation in the neonate; in Crystal RG, West JB, Barnes PJ, Cherniack NS, Weibel ER (eds): The Lung. New York, Raven Press, 1991, pp 1711–1722.
23 Blesa M, Lahiri S, Rashkind W, Fishman AP: Normalization of the blunted ventilatory response to acute hypoxia in congenital cyanotic heart disease. N Engl J Med 1977; 296:237–241.
24 Lahiri S: Peripheral chemoreceptors and their sensory neurons in chronic state of oxygenation; in Fregly MJ, Blatteis C (eds): Adaptation to the Environment (Handbook of Physiol). New York, Oxford University Press, in press.
25 Muligan E, Lahiri S, Storey B: Carotid body O_2 chemoreception and mitochondrial oxidative phosphorylation. J Appl Physiol 1981;51:438–446.
26 Keilin D, Hartree EF: Cytochrome and cytochrome oxidase. Proc R Soc Lond [B] 1939;127:167–191.
27 Lahiri S, Smatresk NJ, Mulligan E: Responses of peripheral chemoreceptors to natural stimuli; in Acker H, O'Regan RG (eds): Physiology of the Peripheral Arterial Chemoreceptors. Amsterdam, Elsevier, 1983, pp 221–256.
28 Müller U, Bühs D, Oehlke-Unterholzner C, Wiemer W: Comparison of carotid chemoreceptor and baroreceptor reactions to anoxia and ischemia; in Pallot D (ed): The Peripheral Arterial Chemoreceptors. London, Croom Helm, 1984, pp 9–16.

Biol Neonate 1994;65:140–144

A. Bairam
B. Hannhart
C. Choné
F. Marchal

Laboratoire de Physiologie,
Faculté de Médecine,
Université de Nancy, France

Effect of Dopamine on Carotid Chemoreceptor Activity in Newborn Kittens

Key Words
Chemoreception
Newborn kitten
Carotid body
Neurotransmitter
Response to hypoxia
Sinus nerve
Dopamine receptors
Glomus cell

Abstract
In newborn kittens, intravenous bolus injections of dopamine may be inhibitory or excitatory to the carotid chemosensory activity. In order to further identify the role of dopaminergic mechanisms on the chemosensory activity in the kitten, 10 anesthetized, paralyzed and artificially ventilated kittens aged from 1 to 21 days were studied. The activity of a few chemoafferent fibers from one carotid sinus nerve was recorded at three levels of Fi_{O_2} in N_2, 21, 8 and 100%, before and during a continuous dopamine infusion at a dose of 10 µg/kg/min. The immediate effect of dopamine usually was a transient inhibition of carotid chemosensory discharge. After 2 min of infusion, the activity had consistently increased from 4.5 ± 0.8 to 8.8 ± 1.4 impulses/s (mean ± SEM, $p < 0.05$) in normoxia. Dopamine also significantly increased the steady state chemosensory response to hypoxia from 24.6 ± 3.7 to 33.4 ± 5.3 impulses/s. Hence, continuous infusion of dopamine has a dual effect on carotid chemoreceptor activity: early inhibition followed by excitation. The excitatory effect enhances the response to hypoxia. These data suggest that the dual effect of dopamine on carotid chemosensory discharge may be related to dopamine concentration in the carotid body.

Introduction

Dopamine may be involved, as a neuromodulator or a neurotransmitter, in the transduction of hypoxia by type I cells in the carotid body and its release and turn over increase during hypoxia [1, 2]. The usual physiological effect of exogenous dopamine in adult mammals is an inhibition of the carotid chemosensory discharge [3–6], although, an excitation

Dr. Aïda Bairam
Laboratoire de Physiologie, Faculté de Médecine
9, avenue de la Forêt de Haye, BP 184
F–54505 Vandœuvre-lès-Nancy Cedex (France)

0006–3126/94/
0654–0140$5.00/0

has occasionally been shown, both in vivo and in vitro [5–7]. The dual effect of dopamine on chemosensory activity might be related to the stimulation of pre- or postsynaptic dopamine receptors that have been identified on glomar cells to carotid chemosensory fiber synapses [8]. Little is known on the relationship between dopaminergic mechanisms and carotid chemosensory activity in the newborn. Mayock et al. [9] found that bolus injection of dopamine has a depressant effect on ventilation which is more important in 1-week-old lambs than in 1-day-old lambs. Dopamine concentration in the carotid body is particularly high at birth [10] and its turn over decreases within the first few hours of life in rat pups [11]. Because of the usual inhibitory effect of exogenous dopamine, it has been suggested that the decrease of dopamine turnover rate was responsible for the maturation of the ventilatory chemoreflex [11]. In newborn kittens, it has been shown that i.v. bolus injection of dopamine mostly inhibited the chemosensory activity during normoxia, while the excitatory effect was predominant during hypoxia [12]. Short term hypoxia is known to increase the release of dopamine from glomus cells [1]. We hypothesized that the increase in dopamine concentration at the level of synaptic cleft by exogenous accumulation of dopamine (continuous infusion) and/or by endogenous release (induced by hypoxia) produce an excitation of the chemosensory discharge. To test this hypothesis, we studied the effect of a continuous infusion of dopamine on chemosensory activity in normoxia and in hypoxia in the kitten.

Material and Methods

Studies were carried out in 10 kittens aged 1–21 days. Their weight ranged from 80 to 350 g. The animal preparation has been described in detail previously [12, 13]. Briefly, the kittens were anesthetized with sodium thiopental (60 mg/kg i.p.) and femoral vessels were cannulated. Rectal temperature was maintained at approximately 38 °C. A tracheostomy was performed and the kittens were artificially ventilated with a respiratory pump and paralyzed with pancuronium bromide (1 mg/kg i.v.). Under a dissecting microscope, the carotid bifurcation was exposed and the carotid sinus nerve was cut at the level of the petrosal ganglion and dissected into fine filaments, in warm mineral oil. The filaments were tested one at the time for neural signal and further divided until one or a few chemoafferents remained. The action potentials were amplified, band pass filtered, fed to a window discriminator and displayed on an oscilloscope and a chart recorder.

Protocol

The carotid chemoreceptor activity was tested by changing the F_{IO_2} in the following sequence: 21%, 8% O_2 in N_2 and 100% O_2. Each gas mixture was held for 2 min. Dopamine was infused at a constant rate of 10 µg/kg/min when the kitten was breathing air. Five minutes after the start of dopamine infusion, the sequence of exposure to the same series of gas was repeated.

Data Analysis

The chemosensory activity expressed as impulses/s was averaged over 10-second epochs. Statistical analysis was done using a two-way analysis of variance to compare carotid sinus nerve activity before and during dopamine infusion. Data were expressed as mean ± SEM. Differences were considered as significant at a p value lower than 0.05.

Results

Chemosensory Response to Continuous Infusion of Dopamine in Normoxia

Figure 1 illustrates a typical response to dopamine in a 4-day-old kitten. After starting dopamine infusion, an inhibition of the chemosensory discharge that lasted for 10 s to 2 min was observed in 5 kittens. This decrease was followed either by a return of the activity to control in 2 kittens, or by a gradual increase in 3 kittens. In 4 kittens, a gradual increase in chemosensory activity was observed from the onset of infusion. In one kitten, the activity did not change. The overall mean chemosen-

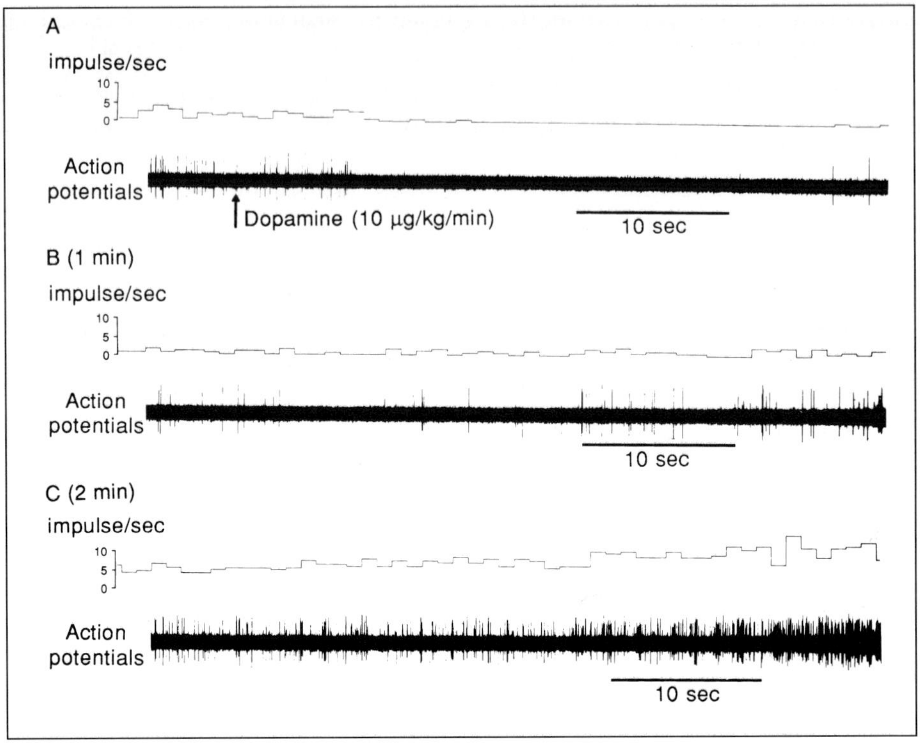

Fig. 1. Carotid chemosensory response to continuous infusion of dopamine in a 4-day-old kitten in normoxia. **A, B** and **C** are continuous. At the onset of dopamine infusion (10 μg/kg/min), there is a clear inhibition of discharge rate (**A**). The activity reappears progressively (**B**), and increases above control value (**C**).

sory activity had reached a steady state within 4 min of the start of dopamine infusion and had increased from a control value of 4.5 ± 0.8 to 8.8 ± 1.4 impulses/s during dopamine ($p < 0.05$). Hence, the late effect of dopamine on chemosensory activity was excitatory.

Response to Hypoxia and Hyperoxia before and after Dopamine

In all kittens, hypoxia induced an increase in chemosensory activity which reached a steady state within 1 min of the onset of hypoxia. Figure 2 shows the steady state chemosensory activity at the three levels of F_{IO_2} before and during dopamine infusion. The

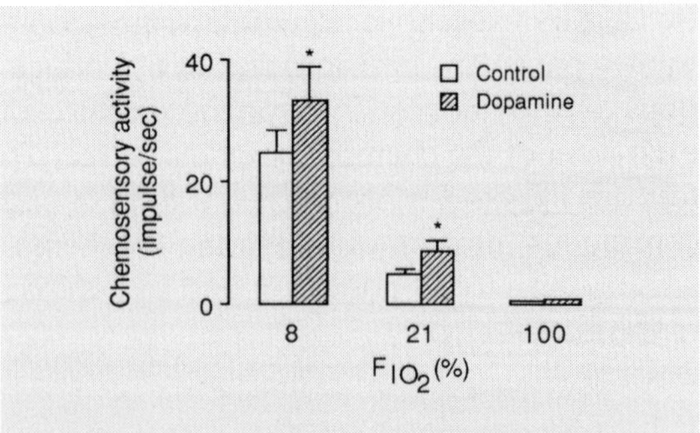

Fig. 2. Carotid chemosensory activity at three F_{IO_2} before and during dopamine infusion (10 μg/kg/min) in 10 kittens. Dopamine significantly increases the steady state activity in normoxia and hypoxia (*$p < 0.05$), but not in hyperoxia.

activity in hypoxia was 24.6 ± 3.7 impulses/s before dopamine and 33.4 ± 5.3 impulses/s after ($p < 0.05$).

Finally, the activity in hyperoxia was similar before and after dopamine (fig. 2).

Discussion

The main findings of this study are that the initial response to continuous infusion of dopamine in normoxia is frequently inhibitory but the late response is excitatory. Furthermore, the chemosensory response to hypoxia is enhanced during dopamine infusion. As reported in a previous study [12], these observations show that the dopaminergic mechanisms are developed in the kitten at birth.

In adult cats, dopamine has been shown to inhibit the chemosensory discharge [3, 14]. In addition to this inhibitory effect, excitation as well as inhibition followed by excitation have been reported after dopamine both in vivo [5] and in vitro [7]. The excitatory effect of dopamine is frequently observed after large bolus injections of dopamine [5]. Hypoxia increases the release and the turnover of dopamine from the carotid body [2]. The depletion of dopamine stores by reserpine inhibits the chemosensory response to hypoxia in the superfused carotid body in vitro [15]. In the kitten, the early response to dopamine infusion was qualitatively similar to that reported in adult cats [3]. However, after several minutes of infusion, excitation of the discharge rate was consistently observed in normoxia and the response to hypoxia was enhanced. These observations suggest that dopamine may be involved to express the carotid chemosensory response to hypoxia.

One hypothesis to explain the inhibitory and the excitatory effect of dopamine is based on the existence of dopamine receptors located on both glomar cells (presynaptically) and sensory nerve endings (postsynaptically) [8]. In the central nervous system, pre- and postsynaptic dopamine receptors have different physiological and pharmacological properties [16]. The presynaptic receptors are autoreceptors that regulate dopamine synthesis and release by a negative feedback mechanism. These receptors have a high affinity for dopamine and their stimulation produces an inhibition of neuronal activity. In contrast, postsynaptic receptors have a lower affinity for dopamine and their stimulation induces an increase in neuronal activity [17]. The inhibitory and the excitatory effects of dopamine on chemosensory discharge may be related to a selective stimulation of pre- and postsynaptic receptors depending on dopamine concentration in the synaptic cleft. Low doses of dopamine may stimulate presynaptic receptors producing an inhibition of the chemoreceptor activity. This effect may be observed at the onset of infusion. High doses of dopamine may stimulate postsynaptic receptors, thus increasing the chemosensory discharge. This mechanism may be involved at a later time of infusion in normoxia, and in hypoxia. In hypoxia, the endogenous release of dopamine may increase its concentration at the synaptic level.

The present study indicates that dopaminergic mechanisms are present in the carotid body of the kitten. It is suggested that the difference in the pattern of response to dopamine compared with adult cats may reflect developmental characteristics of pre- and postsynaptic dopamine receptors in the carotid body.

References

1 Hanbauer I, Hellström S: The regulation of dopamine and noradrenaline in the rat carotid body and its modification by denervation and by hypoxia. J Physiol (Lond) 1978;282:21–34.

2 Péquignot JM, Cottet-Emard JM, Dalmaz Y, Peyrin L: Dopamine and norepinephrine dynamics in rat carotid body during long-term hypoxia. J Autonom Nerv Syst 1987;21:9–14.

3 Lahiri S, Nishino T, Mokashi A, Mulligan E: Interaction of dopamine and haloperidol with O_2 and CO_2 chemoreception in the carotid body. J Appl Physiol 1980;49:45–51.

4 Van Vliet BN, West NH: Functional characteristics of arterial chemoreceptors in an amphibian *(Bufo marinus)*. Respir Physiol 1992;88:113–127.

5 Okajima Y, Nishi K: Analysis of inhibitory and excitatory actions of dopamine on chemoreceptor discharges of carotid body of cat in vivo. Jpn J Physiol 1981;31:695–704.

6 Docherty RJ, McQueen DS: Inhibitory action of dopamine on cat carotid chemoreceptors. J Physiol (Lond) 1978;279:425–436.

7 Zapata P: Effects of dopamine on carotid chemoreceptors and baroreceptors in vitro. J Physiol (Lond) 1975;244:235–251.

8 Mir AK, McQueen DC, Pallot DJ, Nahorski SR: Direct biochemical and neuropharmacological identification of dopamine D-2 receptors in the rabbit carotid body. Brain Res 1984;291:273–283.

9 Mayock DE, Standaert TA, Guthrie RD, Woodrum DE: Dopamine and carotid body function in the newborn lamb. J Appl Physiol 1983;54:814–820.

10 Hervonen A, Kanerva L, Karkala O, Partanen S: Effects of hypoxia and glucocorticoids on the histochemically demonstrable catecholamines of the newborn rat carotid body. Acta Physiol Scand 1972;86:109–114.

11 Hertzberg T, Hellström S, Lagercrantz H, Péquignot JM: Development of the arterial chemoreflex and turnover of carotid body catecholamines in the newborn rat. J Physiol (Lond) 1990;425:211–225.

12 Marchal F, Bairam A, Haouzi P, Hascoet JM, Crance JP, Vert P, Lahiri S: Dual responses of carotid chemosensory afferents to dopamine in the newborn kitten. Respir Physiol 1992;90:173–183.

13 Marchal F, Bairam A, Haouzi P, Crance JP, Di Giulio C, Vert P, Lahiri S: Carotid chemoreceptor response to natural stimuli in the newborn kitten. Respir Physiol 1992;87:183–193.

14 Nishino T, Lahiri S: Effects of dopamine on chemoreflexes in breathing. J Appl Physiol 1981;50:892–897.

15 Leitner LM, Roumy M: Chemoreceptor response to hypoxia and hypercapnia in catecholamine depleted rabbit and cat carotid bodies in vitro. Pflügers Arch 1986;406:419–423.

16 Chesselet MF: Presynaptic regulation of neurotransmitter release in the brain. Neuroscience 1984;12:347–375.

17 Roth RH: Dopamine autoreceptors: Pharmacology, function and comparison with postsynaptic dopamine receptors. Commun Psychopharmacol 1979;3:429–445.

Biol Neonate 1994;65:145–148

Hugo Lagercrantz
Jean-Marc Pequignot
Torbjörn Hertzberg
Hans Holgert
Thomas Ringstedt

Departments of Pediatrics (KS) and Molecular Neurobiology, Karolinska Institute, Stockholm, Sweden;
URA CNRS 1195, Faculté de Médecine Grange-Blanche, Université Claude-Bernard, Lyon, France

Birth-Related Changes of Expression and Turnover of Some Neuroactive Agents and Respiratory Control

Key Words
Fetus
Infant
Respiratory regulation
Dopamine
Noradrenaline
c-fos
Neuropeptides

Abstract
Respiratory movements are partially inhibited before birth and central and peripheral chemoreceptors are probably less sensitive. The transition to continuous breathing might be due to the switch-off of inhibitory neuromodulators and the switch-on of excitatory neuroactive agents. This hypothesis has been explored mainly in rats. One example is dopamine which was found to have a high turnover in carotid bodies in newborn pups prior to decreasing rapidly. It is suggested to inhibit the carotid bodies before birth. In the brain, the noradrenergic system has been found to be activated at birth, possibly promoting neural transmission and arousal. Increased expressions of mRNA for c-fos, tyrosine hydroxylase and some neuropeptides have also been found.

Respiration is episodic and before birth is rather inhibited than stimulated by hypoxia [1]. It becomes more vigorous and continuous immediately after birth, probably due to increased sensory input (cooling), increased PO_2 level, etc. [2]. Hypoxia causes some stimulation of breathing, although the adult response is achieved sometime later. Neuromodulators like adenosine, prostaglandins and placental factors have been postulated to inhibit fetal breathing [2]. The peripheral chemoreceptors have been found to have a lower setpoint before birth [3] possibly inhibited by dopamine, as discussed below.

It can be hypothesized that some excitatory neurotransmitters are not expressed and released before birth. Of particular interest is the general neuronal activation associated with the arousal at birth. This arousal constitutes a major part of the forebrain drive of respiration [4]. Therefore, we have investigated the activation of the locus coeruleus of the rat brain during the perinatal period by measuring noradrenaline turnover. In addition, we have determined mRNA for tyrosine hydroxylase and c-fos, the latter an oncogene which can be studied as a marker of neuronal activity. The expression of some neuropeptide genes, possibly related to respiratory control, are also of interest. Therefore, we will examine the role of some neuroactive agents for the control of respiration during the perinatal pe-

Dr. Hugo Lagercrantz
Department of Pediatrics
Karolinska Hospital
S-171 76 Stockholm (Sweden)

0006–3126/94/
0654–0145$5.00/0

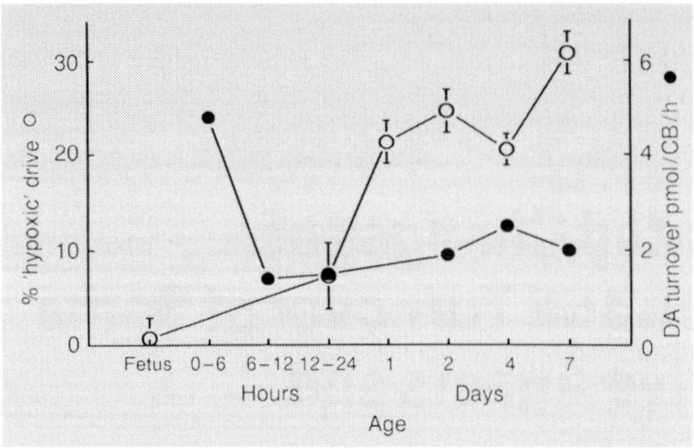

Fig. 1. Development of the hypoxic respiratory drive in relation to dopamine turnover in carotid bodies of newborn rats. When dopamine turnover decreased, the chemoreflex was considerably activated. If the rat pups were made hypoxic, the dopamine turnover was maintained at a high level and the chemoreflex was attenuated. From Crystal RG, West JB et al. (eds): The Lung: Scientific Foundations, 1991.

riod, in particular how some inhibitory neurotransmitters are switched off and excitatory ones switched on around birth.

Dopamine

Dopamine is one of the most abundant neuroactive agents in the peripheral chemoreceptors. Pharmacological and neurophysiological studies have demonstrated that dopamine inhibits chemoreceptor discharge in the adult [5] as well as in the newborn [6]. We have recently proposed that dopamine also inhibits the discharge from the carotid bodies and thus sets their sensitivity at a low PO_2 level [7]. After birth, the environmental PO_2 level is increased which silences the carotid bodies. First, a few days after birth, they adapt to the higher PO_2 level in the extrauterine environment [3]. This change of set point could be related to a decrease of dopamine turnover. The decrease of dopamine turnover could be directly related to the emergence of the peripheral chemoreflex, as studied by a hyperoxic technique according to a modified Dejours test (fig. 1).

The idea that dopamine is responsible for setting the sensitivity of peripheral chemoreceptors around birth was further corroborated by another study [8]: rat pups were delivered in a hypoxic environment and kept at a low oxygen level (12% O_2), simulating the situation in utero. We found that these rat pups sustained their low sensitivity to hypoxia, which could be related to sustained increased dopamine turnover. If the animals were then transferred to air they obtained normal responsiveness to hyperoxia, which could be related to decreased dopamine turnover in their carotid bodies.

Thus, there seems to be a switch-off mechanism of an inhibitory neuroregulator to enhance the respiratory drive soon after birth. According to preliminary studies the expression of the dopamine synthetizing enzyme tyrosine hydroxylase decreases after birth [Holgert et al., pers. commun.]

Noradrenaline

Most of the noradrenergic cell bodies in the brain are clustered in the brain stem, to a large extent in the locus coeruleus (A6), from where terminals project to all parts of the brain [9]. During arousal locus coeruleus is activated and noradrenaline (NA) is diffusely released. This NA hypopolarizes neuronal membranes and promotes neuronal activity in general, thus increasing the 'noise' in the brain.

We have measured the noradrenergic activity by determination of the NA metabolite 3-methoxy-4-hydroxyphenylethylene glycol (MHPG) and its ratio to NA in rat brains during the perinatal period [10]. We found that the MHPG/NA ratio increased about 3-fold from the day before to the day after birth.

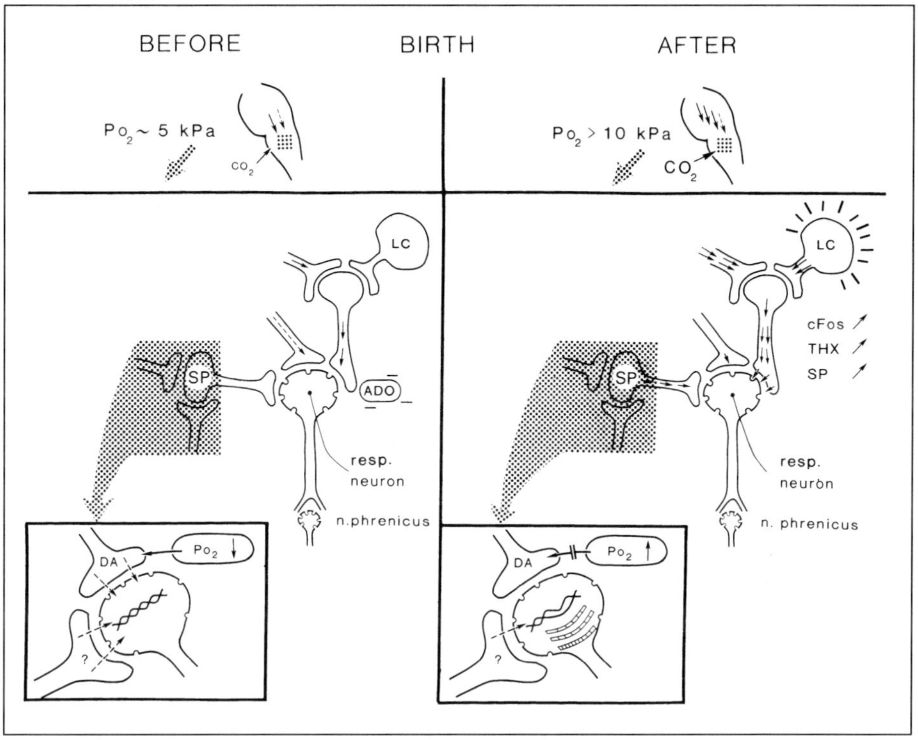

Fig. 2. Before birth breathing is partially inhibited by factors such as low PO_2, adenosine or prostaglandins. There is a sensory deprivation and neuronal activity may be inhibited to some extent. At birth there is an increase in sensory input (e.g. gravity, cooling) which might be responsible for activation of the locus coeruleus (PO_2) and activation of neuronal genes such as c-fos, tyrosine-hydroxylase (TH) and substance P (SP).

This surge of NA turnover in the brain occurred mainly in the 2 h following the breathing of air. The increase of NA turnover was markedly reduced in the cortex after the pups had been breathing a hypoxic gas mixture, while this did not seem to affect NA turnover in the pons medulla. NA turnover was also found to increase in the pons medulla after cooling the rat pups in utero, as compared to controls.

Thus, noradrenergic activity at birth is considerably increased in the brain. Our tentative interpretation is that this reflects the arousal at birth, which is probably of importance for the forebrain drive for breathing. Hypoxia seemed to inhibit the NS turnover in the cortex, possibly related to the general depression of the newborn. On the other hand, cooling stimulated NA turnover. Cooling has been reported to trigger continuous breathing in the fetal sheep and is probably of major importance for stimulating breathing after birth [2].

Furthermore, we have found increased expression of mRNA for c-fos in the cortex and pons medulla of the newborn rats as compared with term fetuses. These findings corroborate the idea of a general neuronal activation at birth. C-fos has also been found to be activated in the central chemoreceptors by CO_2 [11].

Neuropeptides

Neuropeptides like substance P and enkephalins occur in relatively high concentrations in the respiratory nuclei tractus solitarius and might play important roles as neuromodulators of respiratory control [4]. Therefore, we have been interested to determine the expression of some neuropeptides in relation to transitional changes in respiratory control around birth.

Substance P seems to be one of the most abundant neuropeptides in the nucleus tractus solitarius and hypoxic provocation has been shown to increase its release [12]. mRNA encoding for the SP precursor preprotachykinin A was analyzed by Northern blot technique in the respiratory nuclei of the rabbit during the perinatal period [13]. We found a fourfold increase of mRNA for PPT-A in newborn pups which had been breathing air for 2 h as compared with littermates which were sacrificed immediately after cesarean section. Our preliminary studies also indicate increased expression of the SP gene in the pons medulla of newborn rats.

Thus, there seems to be a generally increased expression of excitatory neuroregulators and decrease of inhibitory ones at birth. This switch-on/off of neuroregulatory genes is probably crucial for the transition at birth [14] particularly with regard to respiration (fig. 2).

Acknowledgements

Supported by the Swedish Medical Research Council No. 5234; the Lung and Heart Foundation and Sällskapet Barnavård.

References

1 Dawes GS: The control of fetal breathing and skeletal muscle movements. J Physiol 1984;351:25–37.
2 Adamson SL: Regulation of breathing at birth. J Dev Physiol 1991;15: 45–52.
3 Blanco CE, Dawes GS, Hanson MA, McCooke HB: The response to hypoxia of arterial chemoreceptors in fetal sheep and newborn lambs. J Physiol 1984;351:25–37.
4 Von Euler C: Brain stem mechanisms for generation and control of breathing pattern; in Handbook of Physiology. Baltimore, Williams & Wilkins, 1986, pp 1–67.
5 Llados F, Zapata P: Effects of dopamine analogues and antagonists on carotid body chemosensors in situ. J Physiol 1978;274:487–499.
6 Mayock DE, Standaert TA, Guthrie RD, Woodrum DE: Dopamine and carotid body function in the newborn lamb. J Appl Physiol 1983;54: 814–820.
7 Hertzberg H, Hellström S, Lagercrantz H, Pequignot JM: Development of the arterial chemoreflex and turnover of carotid body catecholamines in the newborn rat. J Physiol 1990;425:211–225.
8 Hertzberg T, Hellström S, Holgert H, Lagercrantz H, Pequignot JM: Ventilatory response to hyperoxia in newborn rats born in hypoxia – Possible relationship to carotid body dopamine. J Physiol 1992;456:645–654.
9 Moore RY, Bloom FE: Central catecholamine neuron systems: anatomy and physiology of the norepinephrine and epinephrine system. Ann Rev Neurosci 1979;2:113–168.
10 Lagercrantz H, Pequignot J, Pequignot JM, Peyrin L: The first breaths of air stimulate noradrenaline turnover in the brain of the newborn rat. Acta Physiol Scand 1992;144:433–438.
11 Sato M, Severinghaus JW, Basbaum AI: Medullary CO_2 chemoreceptor neuron identification by c-fos immunocytochemistry. J Appl Physiol 1992;73:96–100.
12 Lindefors N, Yamamoto Y, Pantaleo T, Lagercrantz H, Brodin E, Ungerstedt U: In vivo release of substance P in the nucleus tractus solitarius increases during hypoxia. Neurosci Lett 1986;69:94–97.
13 Srinivasan M, Yamamoto Y, Persson H, Lagercrantz H: Birth-related activation of preprotachykinin-A mRNA in the respiratory neural structures of the rabbit. Pediatr Res 1991;29:369–371.
14 Lagercrantz H, Srinivasan M: Development and function of neurotransmitter/modulator systems in the brain stem; in Hanson MA (ed): The Fetal and Neonatal Brain Stem. London, Cambridge University Press, 1991, pp 1–20.

Biol Neonate 1994;65:149–155

Henrique Rigatto[a]
Sandra F. Fitzgerald[b]
Maria A. Willis[b]
Chang Yu[b]

[a] Department of Pediatrics, Physiology and Reproductive Medicine, University of Manitoba, Winnipeg, Canada;
[b] Laboratory of Developmental Neurobiology, National Institute of Child Health and Human Development, National Institutes of Health, Bethesda, Md., USA

In Search of the Real Respiratory Neurons: Culture of Medullary Fetal Cells Sensitive to CO_2 and Low pH

Abstract

Although extensively pursued, the real respiratory neurons have remained elusive. We departed from the more conventional physiologic and morphologic methods of system and tissue examination and cultured dissociated fetal rat cells from the areas of the nucleus ambiguus and the nucleus tractus solitarius located within the 2 mm rostral to the obex. Pacemaker-like cells, with a regular single or bursting activity, studied at 3–5 weeks of age, responded to very small pulses of CO_2 (50 ms) and low pH with an increase in spike frequency and a decrease in amplitude. Other irregularly beating or silent cells did not respond or else required very large pulses (>200 ms) to do so. The pacemaker cells also responded to hypoxia induced by administration of sodium hydrosulfite with an increase in spike frequency and amplitude; high oxygen (>600 Torr) and adenosine produced a decrease in electrical activity. Most of these cells were multipolar after staining with antibodies to neuron-specific enolase and fragment C of tetanus toxin. They did not stain for choline acetyltransferase. The results suggest that these cultured cells, expressing a phenotype inherently responsive to CO_2 and low pH, have the characteristics of central respiratory chemoreceptors, and may be involved in the generation of the respiratory rhythm.

Key Words

Respiratory neurons
Respiratory rhythm
Central respiratory control

A histologically well-defined, localized respiratory center has never been found, but neurons known to be vital for respiration occupy the areas of the ventral and dorsal medulla (ventral and dorsal respiratory groups) [1, 3, 4]. The presence of these neurons in various nuclei of the ventral and dorsal medulla have been studied using electrophysiologic [1–3, 5, 6] and immunohistochemical [7, 8] methods applied in vivo and in vitro to fresh tissue preparations [9–12]. With these approaches, the areas of the nucleus ambiguus and adjacencies and that of the tractus solitarius and adjacencies have been identified as important respiratory neuronal pools. Recently, the pre-Bötzinger complex has been suggested as an area that may generate respiratory rhythm in mammals [13].

We decided to modify the traditional strategy of doing electrophysiology in vivo or in large pieces of tissue in vitro, by culturing dissociated fetal cells from the upper medulla in order to discover whether cells with an inherent 'respiratory phenotype' could be found. We reasoned that this phenotype would be typified by cells having (1) a pacemaker-like baseline

Supported by the Medical Research Council of Canada, the Children's Hospital of Winnipeg Research Foundation, and the National Institute of Child Health and Human Development.

Henrique Rigatto, MD
Neonatal Research
RM WR125-735 Notre Dame Avenue
Winnipeg, Manitoba R3L 0L8 (Canada)

pattern of regular beats or bursts of beats; (2) responsiveness to CO_2 and low pH characterized by an increased frequency of beats as compared to baseline. Based on previous study of the location of the central respiratory neuronal pool in rats [5], we selected for dissection slices of the area 2 mm rostral to the obex in the fetal rat (Sprague-Dawley strain) and used a puncture technique [14] or a block dissection [15] to obtain the tissue of interest (fig. 1a, b). The tissue was dissociated and plated on cortex or medulla background [16]. At 3–5 weeks of age, the cells in culture were studied using whole cell patch recording [17, 18].

Tissue for culture, obtained from two slices, 1 mm thick each, rostral to the obex, was minced and treated with trypsin or papain plus DNase. Cells were counted and plated at a concentration of 0.5 to 1 million per dish onto 35-mm diameter culture dishes containing a monolayer of non-neuronal background cells prepared from either cerebral cortex or medulla background [16]. The culture dishes were then placed in an incubator at 37 °C and fed twice weekly with Eagle's minimal essential medium (MEM) containing added horse serum (5%), glucose (600 mg/ 100 ml), $NaHCO_3$ (1.5 g/l), glutamine (2 m*M*), and a number of complex factors [26]. The cultured neurons settled and grew well on top of the prepared non-neuronal substrate, forming a complex network, and were viable at more than 6 weeks of age. Neurons were stained using antibodies against neuron-specific enolase [27], fragment C of tetanus toxin [28] and choline acetyltransferase [29].

Whole patch recordings were carried out in growth medium (PCO_2 51 ± 3 Torr; PO_2 57 ± 10 Torr; pH 7.42 ± 0.03, mean ± SE). The recording pipette had an internal resistance of 3 to 5 MΩ, and contained a recording solution ($KMeSO_4$ 140 m*M*, TEA 1.1 m*M*, $MgCl_2$ 2.0 m*M*, Hepes 10 m*M*, pH 7.2 and osmolarity 310 mosm). A second pipette (3 μm diameter) with similar recording medium equilibrated with high CO_2 (PCO_2 296 ± 42 Torr; pH 6.73 ± 0.06; PO_2 59 ± 4 Torr), and a third pipette equilibrated with any of the remaining compounds were placed at 100 μm from the plasmalemma. Pressure, either maintained or as trains of pulses ranging from 50 to 600 ms duration at a frequency of 1 Hz and a pressure of 2 psi (= 15 kPa), was applied to the back of the perfusion pipettes to produce flow of solution over the cell. The concentrations given are those in the pipette and indicate the upper limit that may actually have reached the cells. Statistical significances were evaluated using analysis of variance (ANOVA) or chi-square analysis.

Randomly chosen neurons originating from areas of the nucleus ambiguus (n = 85) and the tractus solitarius (n = 84) showed one of the following baseline patterns of activity: (1) a regular pacemaker beating activity, single or bursting; (2) an irregular firing pattern or (3) a silent pattern. Pacemaker-like cells were slightly more frequent in the area of the nucleus ambiguus than in the area of the nucleus tractus solitarius (17 vs. 10%), but irregular beating and silent cells were equally distributed in these two areas. Pacemaker cells were uniquely sensitive to CO_2 and low pH, responding usually to pulses of 50 ms with an increase in spike frequency and a decrease in amplitude (fig. 1c, e). Membrane potential usually decreased and input membrane resistance did not change with CO_2 and low pH. These finding suggest that the pacemaker cells (1) work like a current generator in which a major depolarization does not involve an increase in conductance; (2) work as a voltage dependent membrane in which an increase in conductance is masked by the action of CO_2, or (3) work as a combination of these two systems. It is probably safe, though, to assume that CO_2 or low pH does not produce a very large change in conductance.

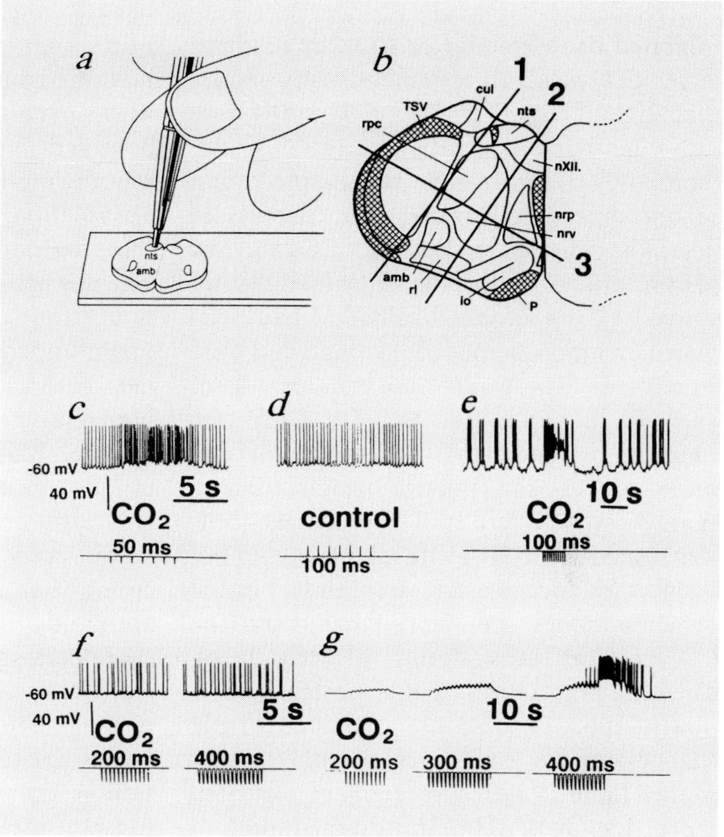

Fig. 1. Dissecting procedure and electrophysiologic responses to pulses of CO_2 and low pH. Top panels: Coronal view of slices, 1 mm thick, taken rostral to the obex. **a** When the puncture technique was used, the nuclei were removed using a special needle as described [14]. **b** When doing block dissection [15] the lateral portion of each side of the slice was removed first (section 1). The diagonal slices having the nucleus ambiguus ventrally and nucleus tractus solitarius dorsally were then removed and divided in the middle (section 2–3). Dissociated cells for the ventral and dorsal areas were plated in different culture dishes. TSV = Spinal trigeminal tract; cul = exterior cuneate nucleus; nts = nucleus tractus solitarius; nXII = hypoglossal nucleus; rpc = parvicellular reticular nucleus; nrv = medullary reticular nucleus, ventral portion; nrp = paramediam reticular nucleus; amb = nucleus ambiguus; rl = lateral nucleus, lateral portion; io = inferior olive; P = area postrema. **c** A single beating pacemaker-like cell responded to a 50-ms pulse of medium equilibrated with CO_2 and low pH with an increase in frequency and in amplitude. Spikes per minute in the pacemaker cells increased from 107 ± 11 at rest to 315 ± 29 during administration of 50-ms pulses of CO_2 ($p = 0.002$). In conjuction with this increased electrical activity, membrane potential decreased from 66 ± 3 to 58 ± 2 mV ($p = 0.02$). Measurements of input membrane resistance, made by applying 0.1 nA, 30–50 ms negative current, during spontaneous electrical activity and during CO_2 administration, were similar (257 ± 14 compared with 260 ± 11 MΩ; $p = 0.8$). Measurements made during administration of tetrodotoxin (TTX) and TTX plus CO_2 were also similar (227 ± 11 compared with 282 ± 9 MΩ; n = 12; $p = 0.7$). **d** Administration of a control solution (same composition but no increase in CO_2) had no effect on the spontaneous electrical activity. **e** A bursting neuron also responded to a pluse of 50 ms with an increase in frequency and a decrease in amplitude; some degree of depolarization was also observed. **f** An irregular beating cell did not respond to pulses of 200 and 400 ms of CO_2. **g** Silent cell showed some depolarization but firing activity was only present with pulses of 400 ms (note: spike amplitude attenuated by chart recorder).

Irregularly beating cells or silent cells were inhibited or insensitive to CO_2, or required larger CO_2 pulses to respond, usually greater than 200 ms (fig. 1f, g). Pacemaker cells were never inhibited or insensitive to CO_2 and, therefore, comprised a well-defined and unique type of cell population. To further determine whether this action of CO_2 and low pH was unique to the cells in the medulla, we studied 12 hippocampal cells that had been plated on hippocampus background and were 21 days old. These cells were primarily silent and usually insensitive to CO_2. Only one silent cell responded to CO_2 but required large pulses of CO_2, the findings being similar to those shown in figure 1g. The pacemaker cells also responded to HCl with an increase in frequency and a decrease in amplitude, but the response was less pronounced than that to the CO_2 solution at a similar pH (fig. 2a, b). These findings suggest that a substantial portion of the CO_2 response is related to pH change and we leave open the question of wether there is a CO_2 component regulated independently of pH [23]. Administration of magnesium chloride ($MgCl_2$) or TTX abolished the resting electrical activity of the pacemaker cells, but their responsiveness to CO_2 remained (fig. 2f, g). These findings further suggest that the CO_2 responsiveness of these regular beating cells is an intrinsic property of the cell.

Neurons responsive to CO_2 and low pH have been observed in fresh slice preparations of the anterior and posterior medulla but their pacemaker-like activity has not been defined [9, 12]. Smith et al. [13] have found pacemaker-like cells in the pre-Bötzinger complex which they suggested are important for breathing pattern generation but the responsiveness of those cells to CO_2 and low pH was not studied. The present findings illustrate that cells within a limited area rostral to the obex not only have a pacemaker-like activity but are uniquely sensitive to CO_2 and low pH. Furthermore, these properties are clearly identified in fetal rat cells even after many weeks in culture. Whether some of these cells observed in the ventral medulla may represent the pre-inspiratory neurons that Arata et al. [10] thought important in the generation of the respiratory pattern remains unknown. The mechanism of action of CO_2 and low pH is unknown but a modified proton channel might underlie this action [24, 25]. Ion channels, such as for Ca^{2+} and Na^+ are also possible candidates and so is the turning off of a K^+ channel [26]. It is also possible that this unique sensitivity is mediated through an entirely different channel.

The response to sodium hydrosulfite consisted of an increase in spike frequency and amplitude; high oxygen tension and adenosine decreased or abolished the spontaneous electrical activity of these cells (fig. 2c–e). Irregular beating cells or silent cells were usually insensitive to these stimuli. The clear distinction in response to these stimuli further reinforce the idea that the pacemaker-like cells are indeed endowed with the characteristics needed for central respiratory chemoreception. The findings are consistent with observations in vivo. For example, the dissociated medullary cell preparation should functionally resemble the medullary center in the fetus after midcollicular brainstem transection [27]. In both situations low O_2 stimulates and high O_2 inhibits 'respiratory' activity. Thus, the inhibitory response to low O_2 previously observed in the intact fetus and newborn [27, 28] is likely not a direct action of low O_2 on the central medullary neurons but may be mediated by the release of an intermediate neurotransmitter. Adenosine which inhibits the pacemaker activity and appears to mediate the response to hypoxia in vivo [29] is a good candidate for this function. Thus, the pacemaker-like cell observed in the present

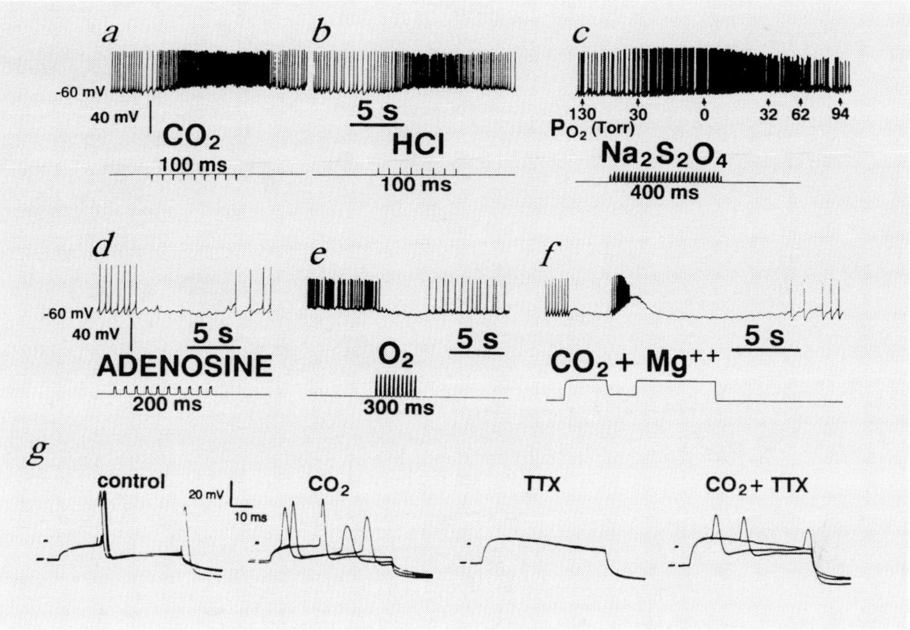

Fig. 2. Responses of the pacemaker cells to medium equilibrated with hydrochloride acid (HCl), sodium hydrosulfite ($Na_2S_2O_4$), adenosine, 100% O_2, $MgCl_2$ and TTX. **a, b** Administration of pulses containing HCl (m*M*) also showed an increase in frequency and a decrease in amplitude but less pronounced than the administration of CO_2 plus low pH (PCO_2 194 Torr in the CO_2 solution; pHs 6.83 in both solutions). **c** A decrease in tissue oxygenation induced by administration of $Na_2S_2O_4$ (m*M*) solution, Sigma) produced an increase in the frequency (78 ± 8 spikes/min to 198 ± 13; p = 0.01) and amplitude (54 ± 4 to 59 ± 3 mV; p = 0.02) of the electrical potentials. Tissue PO_2 was measured using a Clark-Style microoxygen electrode with a 30-μm tip diameter (Diamond General Development Corporation, Product No. 737, Ann Arbor, Mich., USA). **d** Administration of adenosine (9-β-*D*-ribofuranosyladenine μ*M*, Sigma) abolished spontaneous electrical activity. **e** Administration of medium equilibrated with high oxygen (640 Torr) also induced a decrease in cell activity. **f** Synaptic blockade with a continuous pulse of $MgCl_2$ (3 m*M* solution) abolished the spontaneous electrical activity, but this activity resurfaced with administration of CO_2. **g** When the excitability of the cell was tested by measuring the evoked response to a given electrical stimulation there were few evoked potentials at rest (control), many during CO_2 administration, none during tetrodotoxin (TTX 0.5 μ*M*) alone, and many during the administration of TTX plus CO_2.

study appears to have the characteristics needed to function as the cellular unit of the respiratory center network.

The cultured neuronal population in the areas of the nucleus ambiguus and the nucleus tractus solitarius was of heterogeneous morphology including small and large bipolar, pyramidal, and multipolar cells (fig. 3). When stained with antibodies to neuron-specific enolase [20] and fragment C of tetanus toxin [21], the neurons sensitive to CO_2 and low pH did not appear to have a distinct morphologic characteristic, but most were multipolar. The sensitive neurons did not stain for choline acetyltransferase (ChAT) although other neurons in these preparations were immunoreactive for ChAT [22].

In summary, we have isolated and maintained in culture pacemaker-like neurons from the upper medulla in the fetal rat which

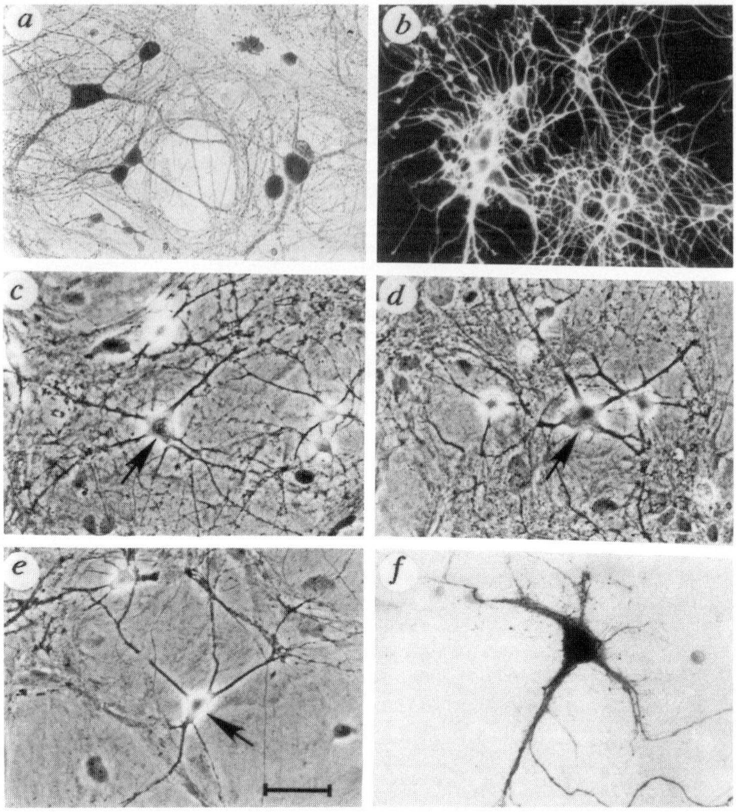

Fig. 3. Dissociated cells from the areas of the nucleus ambiguus (**a**, **c**, **f**) and nucleus tractus solitarius (**b**) plated onto a non-neuronal cellular substate prepared from medulla and maintained in culture for 4 weeks. **a** Immunohistochemistry for neuron-specific enolase confirmed the identity of neurons, which varied in size and number of primary dendrites. **b** Immunofluorescent staining of the neuronal membrane with fragment C of tetanus toxin demonstrated the complexity of the neuronal network. **c**, **d** Neurons (arrows) which were identified electrophysiologically as pacemaker-like cells and responded to elevated CO_2 and low pH with an increase in spike frequency. **e** A neuron which did not respond to applied CO_2. The neurons in **c** and **f** were in the same culture which, after electrophysiologic analysis, was fixed and stained immunohistochemically for choline acetyltransferase (ChAT). None of the CO_2-sensitive cells examined for ChAT immunoreactivity were shown to be cholinergic, although a number of ChAT-immunoreactive neurons (**f**) were present in these cultures. × 200. Bar in **e** represents 50 μm and applies to all panels.

expressed a phenotype inherently responsive to CO_2 and low pH. These characteristics appear to make them prime candidates for central respiratory chemoreception. It is tempting to speculate that these cells may also be involved in a network responsible for the generation of the respiratory rhythm.

Acknowlegements

We thank Miklós Palkovits for help with the tissue sampling. Elaine Neale and Linda Bowers provided assistance with the tissue culture, cell morphology and staining methods. Phillip Nelson provided encouragement and useful criticisms throughout the study.

References

1 Richter DW, Ballantyne D: A three phase theory about the basic respiratory pattern generator; in Schlafke WE, Koepchen HD, See WR (eds): Central Neurone Environment, Berlin, Springer, 1983, pp 164–174.
2 Feldmann JL, Smith JC: Cellular mechanisms underlying modulation of breathing pattern in mammals. Ann NY Acad Sci 1989;563:114–130.
3 Cohen MI: Neurogenesis of respiratory rhythm in the mammal. Physiol Rev 1979;59:1105–1173.
4 Merril EG: Where are the real respiratory neurons? Fed Proc 1981;40: 2389–2394.
5 Saether K, Hilaire G, Monteau R: Dorsal and ventral respiratory groups of neurons in the medulla of the rat. Brain Res 1987;419:87–96.
6 Etzure K, Manabe M, Yamada H: Distribution of medullary respiratory neurons in the rat. Brain Res 1988;455:262–270.
7 Ellenberger HH, Feldman JF: Subnuclear organization of the lateral tegmental field of the rat. I. Nucleus ambiguus and ventral respiratory group. J Comp Neurol 1990;294: 202–211.
8 Sales N, Riche D, Roques BP, Denavit-Saubie M: Localization of μ- and δ-opioid receptors in cat respiratory areas: An autoradiographic study. Brain Res 1985;344:382–386.
9 Dean JB, Bayliss DA, Erickson JT, Lawing WL, Millhorn DE: Depolarization and stimulation of neurons in nucleus tractus solitarii by carbon dioxide does not require chemical synaptic input. Neuroscience 1990; 36:207–216.
10 Arata A, Onimaru H, Homma I: Respiration-related neurons in the ventral medulla of newborn rats in vitro. Brain Res Bull 1990;24:599–604.
11 Dekin MS, Richerson GB, Getting PA: Thyrotropin-releasing hormone induces rhythmic bursting in neurons of the nucleus tractus solitarius. Science 1985;229:67–69.
12 Jarolimek V, Misgeld U, Lux HD: Neurons sensitive to pH in slices of the rat ventral medulla oblongata. Pflügers Arch 1990;416:247–253.
13 Smith JC, Ellenberger HH, Ballanyi K, Richter DW, Feldmann JL: Pre-Bötzinger complex: A brainstem region that may generate respiratory rhythm in mammals. Science 1991; 254:726–729.
14 Palkovits M, Brownstein MJ: Maps and Guide for Microdissection of the Rat Brain. New York, Elsevier, 1987, plate 198.
15 Yu WA: Dissection of motor nuclei of trigeminal, facial, and hypoglossal nerve from fresh rat brain; in Shahar A, de Vellis J, Vernadakis A, Haber B (eds): A Dissection and Tissue Culture Manual of the Nervous System. New York, Liss, 1989, pp 30–39.
16 Neale EA, Fitzgerald SC, Bowers LM, Yu C, Fields RD, Nelson PG: Muticompartment cell cultures for studies of neuronal interaction; in Conn PM (ed): Methods in Neurosciences. San Diego, Academic Press, 1991, vol. 4, pp 321–349.
17 Ransom BR, Neale E, Henkart M, Bullock PN, Nelson PG: Mouse spinal cord in cell culture. I. Morphology and intrinsic neuronal electrophysiologic properties. J Neurophysiol 1977;40:1132–1150.
18 Fields RD, Yu C, Nelson PG: Calcium network activity and the role of NMDA channels in synaptic plasticity in vitro. J Neurosci 1991;11: 134–146.
19 Fitzgerald SC: Dissociated spinal cord-dorsal root ganglia cultures on plastic tissue culture dishes and glass coverslips and wells; in Shahar A, de Vellis J, Vernadakis A, Haber B (eds): A Dissection and Tissue Culture Manual of the Nervous System. New York, Liss, 1989, pp 219–222.
20 Brenneman DE, Neale EA, Foster GA, d'Autremont SW, Westbrook GL: Nonneuronal cells mediate neurotrophic action of vasoactive intestinal peptide. J Cell Biol 1987;104: 1603–1610.
21 Neale EA, Habig WH, Schrier BK, Bergey GK, Bowers LM, Koh J: Applications of tetanus toxin for structure-function studies in neuronal cell cultures; in Nistico G, Bizzini B, Bytchenko G, Triau R (eds): Eighth International Conference on Tetanus. Rome, Pythagora Press, 1989, pp 58–65.
22 Wang FZ, Nelson PG, Fitzgerald SC, Hersh LB, Neale EA: Cholinergic function in cultures of mouse spinal cord neurons. J Neurosci Res 1990;25:312–323.
23 Eldrige FL, Kiley JP, Milhorn DE: Respiratory responses to medullary hydrogen ion changes in cats: different effects of respiratory and metabolic acidoses. J Physiol (Lond) 1985;358:285–297.
24 Krishtal OA, Pidoplichko VI: A receptor for protons in the nerve cell membrane. Neuroscience 1980;5: 2325–2327.
25 Konnerth A, Lux HD, Morad M: Proton-induced transformation of calcium channel in chick dorsal root ganglion cells. J Physiol (Lond) 1987;386:603–633.
26 Hille B: Ionic Channels of Excitable Membranes. Sunderland, Sinauer Associates Inc., 1984, pp 113–118.
27 Dawes GS, Gardner WM, Johnston BM, Walker DW: Breathing in fetal lambs: The effect of brain stem section. J Physiol (Lond) 1983;335: 535–553.
28 Rigatto H, Brady JP: Periodic breathing and apnea in preterm infants. II. Hypoxia as a primary event. Pediatrics 1972;50:219–228.
29 Runold M, Lagercrantz H, Prabaakar HR, Fredholm BB: Role of adenosine in hypoxic ventilatory depression. J Appl Physiol 1989;67: 541–546.

Biol Neonate 1994;65:156–159

James J. Filiano

Department of Pediatrics (Intensive Care/Neurology), Children's Hospital at Dartmouth, Dartmouth Hitchcock Medical Center, Lebanon, N.H., USA

Arcuate Nucleus Hypoplasia in Sudden Infant Death Syndrome: A Review

Key Words

Arcuate nucleus
Ventral medulla
Sudden infant death syndrome
Respiratory chemosensors
Central respiratory control
Apnea
Ondine's curse
Sleep apnea
Brainstem development
Cerebellum

Abstract

Abnormalities in central ventilatory control during sleep and/or impaired arousal have been reported in some infants who subsequently die of SIDS. Hypothetically, these abnormalities may result from dysfunction of the ventral medullary rim, considered to be an integrative site for cardioventilatory control on the basis of research in animals. This paper summarizes comparative neuroanatomic evidence from a previously published study showing that the human medullary arcuate nucleus is homologous to neurons in the cat which participate in chemosensory/autonomic integrative processes of the ventral medullary rim. Next, it summarizes a study of serially or extensively sectioned medullae of 41 SIDS and 27 controls which identified 2 SIDS victims with isolated hypoplasia of the arcuate nucleus confirmed by three-dimensional reconstructions and volume measurements. The volume of the right arcuate nucleus in the SIDS case was 0.7 mm^3, compared to a range of 3.4–26.3 mm^3 (median 5 mm^3) in 3 infant controls. On the basis of pre-cerebellar and other anatomic connections of the arcuate nucleus and of neurons in homologous positions in animals, arcuate hypoplasia may lead to death by dyssynergy between the cerebellum's influence on cardioventilation and the way this influence is integrated with chemosensation and arousal during sleep and hypercarbia during a critical developmental period.

Introduction

Epidemiologic studies link SIDS with sleep periods, leading to the premise that SIDS occurs during sleep or sleep/waking transitions. This association, combined with data indicating impaired autonomic function and/or arousal in infants who suffer apparent life-threatening events or subsequently die of SIDS is the basis of the hypothesis that SIDS is caused by a defect in state-modulated central regulation of cardioventilatory function [1–6]. An anatomic site relevant to this hypothesis is located near the ventral medullary surface: although the function of each cell population is controversial, neurons and glial along the ventrolateral, ventral, and ventromedial medullary surface and the ventral raphe are generally considered to have an integrative role in autonomic function, ventilation, chemosensitivity, and arousal [7, 11]. We refer to this region collectively as the 'ven-

James J. Filiano, MD
Department of Pediatrics (Intensive Care/Neurology)
Children's Hospital at Dartmouth
Dartmouth Hitchcock Medical Center, 1 Medical Center Drive
Lebanon, NH 03756 (USA)

0006–3126/94/
0654–0156$5.00/0

tral medullary rim' (VMR). Potentially, a subset of SIDS may be caused by dysfunction of the VMR. The following is a summary of two studies investigating this hypothesis.

The Arcuate Nucleus

Experiments in cats and in medulla slice preparations identify neuronal and glial populations in the VMR which respond to carbon dioxide and hydrogen ion and have been termed the respiratory chemosensitive fields (RCFs) [7–11]. In an attempt to find homologous cell populations in the human infant, we compared cat and human infant medullae stained by both hematoxylin and eosin/Luxol fast blue and cresyl violet stains: we found that the size, shape, staining characteristics, distance from the pial surface, and position in the medulla of neurons of the human arcuate nucleus (ARC) were nearly identical to those of a population of neurons in the cat medulla which are considered components of the cat RCFs [10]. ARC neurons are small, round or multipolar, with eccentric nuclei, prominent nucleoli, and indistinct Nissl substance. They are located in a large collection in fibrillary neuropil at the surface surrounding the ventromedian sulcus contiguous with the n. raphe pallidus and extend in clusters superficial to the pyramidal tract, at the ventrolateral sulcus, and adjacent to the n. reticularis lateralis ventralis or n. paragigantocellularis lateralis. The cytoarchitectonic homology was confirmed by three-dimensional computer reconstructions.

In experimental animals, neurons in locations homologous to the human ARC have been called by a variety of names depending on the species, but most commonly the ventral (small cell) division of the n. raphe pallidus, or superficial neurons of the n. paragigantocellularis lateralis [11]. Such neurons connect with forebrain, brain stem, and spinal cord regions vital to cardioventilation and arousal; they synthesize and respond to neurotransmitters/modulators which mediate cardioventilation and autonomic events [7–11]. Thus, generalizing from animal data, the human ARC may contribute to circuitry which mediates cardioventilation. In particular, the precerebellar connections of the ARC may be an anatomic substrate by which the cerebellum contributes to autonomic regulation, linking the VMR to rostral regions and parts of the cerebellum involved in ventilation and autonomic regulation, e.g. the anterior lobe, paramedian lobule, posterior vermis, and fastigial nucleus [1, 11]. Supporting these generalizations are reports of ventilatory disturbance in cases of ARC lesions in humans, and lesions in the ventrolateral medulla and cerebellar system associated with autonomic disturbances and SIDS [11].

Arcuate Nucleus Hypoplasia in SIDS

Based on the potential role of the ARC in ventilatory and autonomic regulation, we tested a hypothesis that anatomic deficiency of the ARC is associated with SIDS [11]. We examined (blinded) serially sectioned medullae of SIDS and controls from an infant brain stem database [10–13]. SIDS was defined as the sudden death of an infant under 1 year of age which remains unexplained after a thorough case investigation, including performance of a complete autopsy, examination of the death scene, and review of the clinical history [14]. Controls were infants whose death was sudden or anticipated, and in whom the autopsy established a cause of death. Some cases were hemisected at autopsy, the right half fixed in formalin, embedded in paraffin, and serially sectioned at 20 μm; nonhemisected brain stems were processed similarly.

The brain stems of 41 SIDS (median age: 12 postnatal weeks; range: 3–43 postnatal weeks) and 27 controls (median age: 15 postnatal weeks; range: 2–53 postnatal weeks) were examined. [see 11 for list of causes of death in the control group]. Every tenth section was stained with hematoxylin and eosin/Luxol fast blue. The amount of ARC was scored visually as abundant, present, or nearly/totally absent. Two cases were found with an almost total absence of the ARC. After breaking the code at the end of the survey, we found that they were SIDS victims. Their clinical histories and autopsy findings have been reported [11], and cannot be distinguished from other SIDS cases in which the ARC was intact: SIDS 1 was a 4.54 kg- (25%), 10-week-old white boy; SIDS 2 was a 5.45 kg (50%), 11-week-old white girl. The few ARC neurons present in these 2 cases were cytologically well differentiated, and immunostaining for glial fibrillary acid protein did not reveal gliosis in the ARC. There were no other abnormalities in the microscopic examination of the brains of these 2 cases; thus, the infants appeared to have an isolated hypoplasia of the ARC.

Across the full study population of 68 brain stems, we found considerable variability in the relative amounts of the ARC between cases, and considerable variability in the amount of ARC from section to section in each case [11]. Therefore, to confirm that the observation of ARC hypoplasia was not a sampling artifact, the medullae of SIDS 1 with ARC hypoplasia and 3 controls with histologically normal brains were studied by three-dimensional reconstruction and volumetric measurements [see 11–13 for methods]. Control 1 was a 50-postconceptional-weeks-old white boy with partial DeGeorge syndrome, truncus arteriosus, and postoperative death following cardiac surgery; control 2 was a 50-postconceptional-weeks-old black male who died suddenly with acute pulmonary infection; and control 3 was 62-postconceptional-weeks-old white boy who died with pulmonary complications of metastatic neuroblastoma. Volume of the right ARC from SIDS 1 was 0.7 mm^3 compared to a range of 3.4–26.3 mm^3 (median 5 mm^3) in the controls. Thus, although the volumetric measurements confirmed the wide variability in the amount of ARC, it nevertheless confirmed the dramatic hypoplasia of the ARC in SIDS 1: the volume of the right ARC from SIDS 1 was 5–37 times smaller than that of the 3 controls. SIDS 2 was not reconstructed because a 2 mm portion of midmedulla was not obtainable. In this case, 43 step-sections through three available medullary blocks were compared, section by section, with corresponding sections from each of the three reconstructed control medullae. In SIDS 2, the ARC was markedly diminished or absent in all 43 sections examined.

Conclusion

This paper summarized two previously published studies: a comparative anatomy study which gave evidence that the human ARC is involved in cardioventilatory control, and a study revealing 2 cases of ARC hypoplasia in a database of 41 SIDS victims (5%), suggesting that ARC hypoplasia is associated with a subset of SIDS. The cause of ARC hypoplasia in the 2 SIDS victims is unknown, but, based on the fetal development of the ARC, a genetic or toxic insult to the regulation of ARC neuron number during the first 16 weeks of pregnancy must be considered [11]. Based on the anatomic connections of the ARC and those of neurons with homologous locations in animals, we postulate that ARC hypoplasia leads to death by causing cardioventilatory dyssynergy and impaired arousal responses to hypercarbia during sleep, including mechanisms which maintain airway patency. This may be most likely to occur during a critical period in the development of autonomic and ventilatory control [see 'The Triple Risk Model of SIDS' in this issue p. 194 and 1]. ARC dysfunction, but without hypoplasia, may be more common in SIDS, however, with these 2 cases representing the severe end of a spectrum of ARC pathology. Alternatively, the markedly reduced volume of ARC may represent biologic variability with no pathophysiologic significance, or an epiphenomenon of some other disturbance in SIDS, and not, of itself, the cause of death. Ultimately, ARC hypoplasia may not be restricted to SIDS deaths, but may be found in other disorders where it may contribute to a victim's vulnerability to die suddenly. To determine which is the truth, further studies are needed, using serial sections, or at least 10 step-sections through the medulla. These studies must establish the normal range of ARC volumes in a large database of autopsied infants in the SIDS age range in order to determine the incidence of ARC hypoplasia in SIDS, and to correlate ARC findings with other morphologic and/or chemical abnormalities in SIDS victims.

Acknowledgements

This work was supported by grants from the Hearst Foundation, National Sudden Infant Death Syndrome Foundation, National Institute of Child Health and Human Development (RO1-HD20991), and Children's Hospital Mental Retardation Core Grant (P30-HD18655). John Stevens, PhD, and Kristen Harris, PhD, provided ICAR 80.8 from ISG Technologies for the brain stem reconstructions. Mrs. Marie Valdes-Dapena, John E. Smialeck, and Alfred Steinschneider developed the autopsy database of SIDS and control cases for the study of tissue markers of hypoxia in SIDS. Dr. Hannah C. Kinney provided the brainstem sections, skeptical critiquc and friendship.

References

1 Kinney HC, Filiano JJ, Harper RM: The neuropathology of the sudden infant death syndrome. J Neuropathol Exp Neurol 1991;51:115–126.
2 Hunt CE: Impaired arousal from sleep: Relationship to sudden infant death syndrome. J Perinatol 1989;9: 184–187.
3 Shannon DC, Kelly DH: SIDS and apnea of infancy; in Chernick V, Kendig EI, (eds): Disorders of the Respiratory Tract in Children. Philadelphia, Saunders, 1990, pp 939–957.
4 Newman NM, Trinder JA, Philips KA, Cruickshank J: Arousal deficit: mechanism of the sudden infant death syndrome. Aust Paediatr J 1989;22:111–116.
5 Harper RM: State-related physiological changes and risk for the sudden infant death syndrome. Aust Paediatr J 1986;(suppl):55–58.
6 Matthews T, Dunne K: End-tidal carbon dioxide levels and the sudden infant death syndrome. Irish Med J 1986;79:212–214.
7 Millhorn DE, Eldridge FL: Role of ventrolateral medulla in regulation of respiratory and cardiovascular systems. J Appl Physiol 1986;61: 1249–1263.
8 Nattie EE: Central respiratory chemoreceptors; in Haddad GG, Farber JP (eds): Developmental Neurobiology of Breathing. New York, Marcel Decker, 1991, pp 341–371.
9 Hilton SM, Marshall JM, Timms RJ: Ventral medullary relay neurones in the pathway from the defense areas of the cat and their effect on blood pressure. J Physiol 1983; 345:149–166.
10 Filiano JJ, Choi JC, Kinney HC: Candidate cell populations for respiratory chemosensitive fields in the human infant medulla. J Comp Neurol 1990;293:448–465.
11 Filiano JJ, Kinney HC: Arcuate nucleus hypoplasia in the sudden infant death syndrome. J Neuropathol Exp Neurol 1992;51:394–403.
12 Kinney HC, Meagher CC, Simons JE, Matthysse SW: Volumetric sampling strategies for heterogeneous brainstem nuclei. J Neuropathol Exp Neurol 1989;48:223–244.
13 Kinney HC, Filiano JJ, Brazy JE, Burger PC, Sidman RL: Congenital apnea with medullary and olivary hypoplasia: a pathologic study with computer reconstructions. Clin Neuropathol 1989;8:163–173.
14 Willinger M, James LS, Catz C: Defining the sudden infant death syndrome (SIDS): Deliberations of an expert panel convened by the National Institute of Child Health and Human Development. Pediatr Pathol 1991;11:677–684.

Biol Neonate 1994;65:160–165

Gabriel G. Haddad
Chun Jiang

Department of Pediatrics,
Section of Respiratory Medicine
(Laboratory of Respiratory
Neurobiology), Yale University
School of Medicine, New Haven,
Conn., USA

Mechanisms of Neuronal Survival during Hypoxia: ATP-Sensitive K^+ Channels

Abstract

There has been an explosion in our understanding of how nerve cells in mammals respond to O_2 deprivation and what are the mechanisms involved in nerve cell injury or survival. This is due to the development of new approaches, techniques and the clinical importance of brain ischemia and hypoxia. Recently, we have focussed on some issues pertaining to brain hypoxia in the newborn and adult. We have demonstrated that during anoxia intracellular K^+ decreases significantly in nerve cells and that this K^+ efflux is mediated by K^+ channels that are sensitive to ATP. We have preliminary evidence that the activation of these channels attenuates the anoxia-induced depolarization in medullary neurons and can play a role in cell survival during anoxia. Further, we have characterized the distribution of these receptors/channels complexes in the CNS of the rat and in an anoxia-resistant animal: the turtle. These channels are present mainly in the cortex, substantia nigra and the cerebellum. Whole cell recordings (dissociated cells) established that these channels are postsynaptic in nature in medullary neurons. Single-channel recordings from our laboratory and those of others have started to reveal the intricacies of the regulation of these channels in excitable cells in general and in nerve cells in particular.

Key Words

Ion channels
Biophysical properties
Anoxia
Maturation
Excitable cells
Nucleotides

Introduction

In the past decade, an enormous number of studies have been performed on the response and sensitivity of central neurons (brain stem and more rostral areas) to hypoxia [1–6]. These experiments have shown that mammalian neurons are exquisitely sensitive to the lack of O_2, that neonatal neurons are much more resistant to hypoxia and that some lower vertebrates (e.g. fresh-water turtles, goldfish) and invertebrates are extremely insensitive to O_2 deprivation to the extent that they can tolerate an environment devoid of O_2 for hours, days and even weeks and months [7–11]. During the past decade, we have also started to understand the ways and the mechanisms that can lead to nerve cell injury [1, 6, 12]. For example, it is recognized that glutamate release from nerve cells during anoxia can bind to a number of receptors, open cation channels, and induce currents carried by Na^+ and Ca^{2+}, leading to cell damage and death [1, 12]. However, it is also clear that glutamate is only one component of a very complex situation at the level of the single cell that is exposed to lack of O_2. Indeed, there is a vast number of potential mechanisms that can be activated or inactivated during this

Gabriel G. Haddad, MD
Pediatrics – Respiratory Medicine
Yale University School of Medicine
333 Cedar Street, Fitkin Bldg., Rm. 506
New Haven, CT 06520 (USA)

stress and these mechanisms may have a protective or a deleterious effect to neurons [6]. A number of reviews exist addressing some of these issues and questions [6, 12, 13]. In this paper, we will review the evidence for the role of ATP-sensitive K^+ channels during anoxia in the CNS by focussing mostly on this rather recently discovered K^+ channel [6, 14–16].

K^+ Efflux and Channels during Hypoxia

We and others have shown that extracellular K^+ (K_o^+) increases during O_2 deprivation [4–6, 17–20]. We have recently demonstrated that this increase in K_o^+ depends on age, grey vs. white matter, CNS region, tissue temperature and presence or absence of glucose and severity of O_2 deprivation [4, 5, 19, 20]. However, questions concerning the source of K^+ and the mechanisms of release have remained unclear. Studies from our laboratory have provided some insight into these issues [19, 20]. For example, using ion-selective microelectrodes and brainstem slices, we have measured intra- and extracellular K^+ concentrations in hypoglossal neurons during anoxia [19, 20]. Extracellular recordings showed that a short period of anoxia (4 min) induced a major increase in K_o^+ in the XII nucleus of adult rats [4, 5, 19, 20]. Intracellular recordings in XII neurons showed a substantial decrease in K_i^+ during anoxia [19]. These results strongly suggested that K^+ is lost from XII neurons during anoxia. Although the extracellular space (ECS) shrank by ~50% during anoxia, the possibility that the increase in K_o^+ and decrease in K_i^+ were mainly caused by shrinkage of the ECS and swelling of intraneuronal space was excluded because the changes in K_i^+ and K_o^+ during anoxia were relatively very large [19, 20].

To study the mechanisms by which K^+ is lost from XII neurons, we used several pharmacologic blockers. High concentration of ouabain (10 m*M*) and strophanthidin (80 μ*M*) substantially increased K_o^+ from baseline. Of interest is that Na-K ATPase blockers did not abolish an additional anoxia-induced increase in K_o^+, suggesting that mechanisms other than Na^+-K^+-adenosine triphosphatase inhibition were also responsible for the anoxia-induced K^+ leakage [19, 20]. Glibenclamide and tolbutamide, two specific ATP-sensitive K^+ channel blockers, prevented half of the K^+ loss usually seen during anoxia in a dose-dependent response. Other K^+ channel blockers (e.g. apamin) had no effect. This suggested that anoxia-induced K^+ loss from XII neurons is related to the activation of an ATP-sensitive process. Therefore, we concluded that during anoxia, XII neurons lose their cytosolic K^+, which substantially contributes to the increase in K_o^+; and that the loss of neuronal intracellular K^+ is mediated to a large degree by the activation of ATP-sensitive K^+ channels in XII neurons.

^{3}H-Glibenclamide Autoradiography

In order to ascertain the existence and localization of ATP-sensitive channels in the CNS, we used autoradiographic techniques and ^{3}H-glibenclamide and examinded binding density and affinity of these sites at a number of CNS levels. Since the adult turtle is resistant to anoxia, we also compared the rat to the turtle brain sulfonylurea receptor distribution [21]. In all three animal groups (newborn rat, adult rat, adult turtle), specific glibenclamide binding was saturable. Scatchard plots were curvilinear in the rat, thus suggesting that glibenclamide binds to two types of sites, i.e. high- and low-affinity sites. Turtle brain tissue showed evidence of one binding site only. We also found that the distribution of glibenclamide binding sites was heterogeneous in the adult rat CNS with a higher density in rostral than in caudal regions. The highest binding densities were seen in the cortex and substantia nigra. Intermediate densities were observed in the basal ganglia and the medullary hypoglossal nucleus. There was a low density in most areas of the hypothalamus, brain stem, and spinal cord. Compared with the adult rat, the newborn had a very homogeneous distribution of binding sites and densities were very low throughout the CNS; the level of binding density was even lower and in some regions undetectable in the adult turtle. Sulfonylurea receptors increase in number postnatally in the rat since binding density increases and the K_d in the newborn rat is similar to that in the adult rat. We believe that K_{ATP} channels and sulfonylurea receptors are poorly developed in the turtle and develop mostly after birth in the rat perhaps when the need for such channels arises [21].

Physiologic Role of K_{ATP} Channels: Whole Cell and Single-Channel Recordings

These previous physiologic and autoradiographic studies on brain stem slices and sections have suggested that K_{ATP} channels are present in CNS neurons and that they are activated during anoxia in XII neurons [6]. To obtain additional evidence for their presence and their physiologic role, we performed studies in dissociated neurons and applied patch clamp techniques using the whole-cell configuration. We found that the majority of XII cells studied have measurable glibenclamide-sensitive outward currents. In addition, as expected if these channels were expressed on XII neuronal membranes, cromokalim, a potent activator of these channels increases the outward currents and decreases the negative holding current. Thus, we have provided direct evidence for the presence of K_{ATP} currents on postsynaptic membranes of XII neurons. However, in rat hippocampal pyramidal neurons, these channels seem to be localized on presynaptic membranes [3], although direct evidence is lacking.

Based on the previous studies from our laboratory including those done on dissociated neurons and those of others [6], it is now clear that there are ATP-sensitive K^+ channels in the CNS and that these play a major role in anoxia [6, 20]. One important and interesting series of experiments that we performed in XII neurons in the slice attest to their crucial role [19, 20]. These experiments have shown us that: (1) XII neurons depolarize more during anoxia in the presence of glibenclamide than during control or baseline recordings and, importantly; (2) they did not recover from O_2 lack when exposed to the stress for the same amount of time in the presence of the sulfonylurea ligand. Hence, we believe that the activation of these ATP-sensitive K^+ channels (i.e. in the absence of glibenclamide) is beneficial during anoxia [19, 20].

In order to understand further the inherent regulation of these ATP-sensitive channels, we have started recording from excised patches' single channels. Although brain stem neurons, especially XII, contain these K^+ channels, we opted to study them from membranes containing a high density of such channels in order to increase the yield of finding those that are sensitive to ATP. Preliminary results (fig. 1) showed that patches from neurons in the substantia nigra are rich in these channels and that a high percentage of outward currents with reversal potential for K^+ are very sensitive to ATP and ADP.

Expression of K_{ATP} Channels in Various Tissues: Potential Roles

ATP-sensitive K^+ channels (K_{ATP}) were first described in cardiac myocytes [14], and later found in almost all excitable tissues [6,

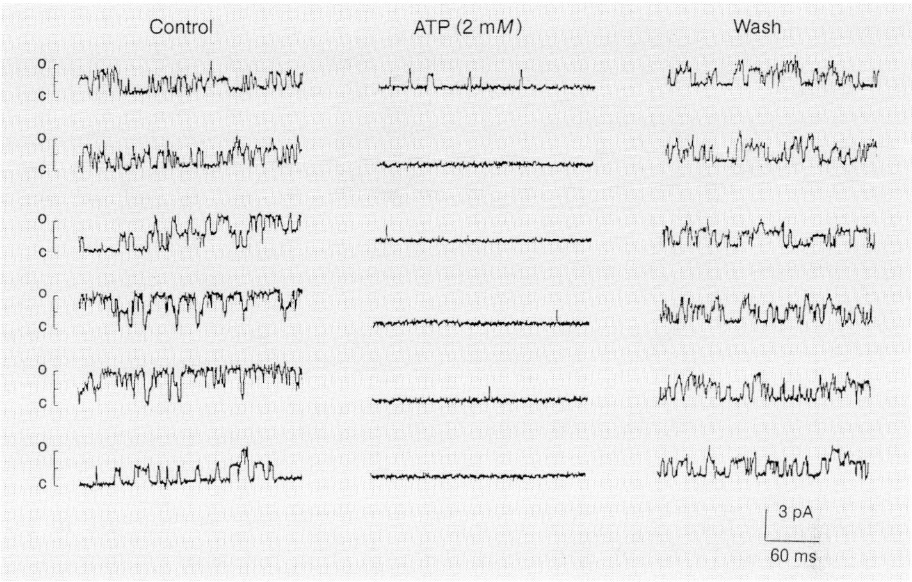

Fig. 1. ATP-sensitive K^+ channels recorded from a freshly dissociated substantia nigra neuron. Excised patch (inside-out) was obtained with bath solution containing (in m*M*) 150 KCl, 10 HEPES and 10-*D*-glucose and pipette solution containing 150 choline chloride, 3 KCl, 1 $CaCl_2$, 1 $MgCl_2$, 10 HEPES and 25-*D*-glucose. Two channels are active at a holding potential of –10 mV (left panel). Single activity was almost totally suppressed when the patch was perfused with the same bath solution containing 2 m*M* ATP (middle panel). Channel activity fully recovered after returning to the bath solution (right panel). o = Channel opening; c = closing. From Jiang and Haddad [unpubl. observations].

14–16]. There are only a few recent reports on K_{ATP} channels in central neurons [6, 16].

These channels are normally inhibited by physiological levels of ATP [6, 14–16]. A decrease in cytosolic ATP concentration, such as during hypoxia or hypoglycemia, opens these channels and leads to membrane hyperpolarization [6, 14, 15, 19–23]. This property of K_{ATP} channels provides a direct link between cellular intermediary metabolism and membrane excitability, through specific biophysical involvement of plasma membranes. It is interesting to note that the regulation of ATP-sensitive K^+ channels may not be only through ATP levels (as stated above) but through levels of ADP or AMP (e.g. energy charge) or via changes of other regulators such as intracellular pH [14, 22, 24]. This diversity in regulators may allow cells to better match cell-specific metabolic alterations during anoxia to these K^+ channels. For example, the rate of ATP drop with anoxia will vary with various types of cells within the CNS or among various types of excitable cells in mammals.

K_{ATP} channels play an important role in the functioning of excitable cells in general. For example, it is believed that insulin secretion from pancreatic β-cells [6, 14] and dilatation of vascular smooth muscles are based on the activation of K_{ATP} channels [6]. Although the critical role of these channels in central neurons is not yet totally clear [6], our recent studies detailed above have suggested that activation of K_{ATP} channels during anoxia may be of

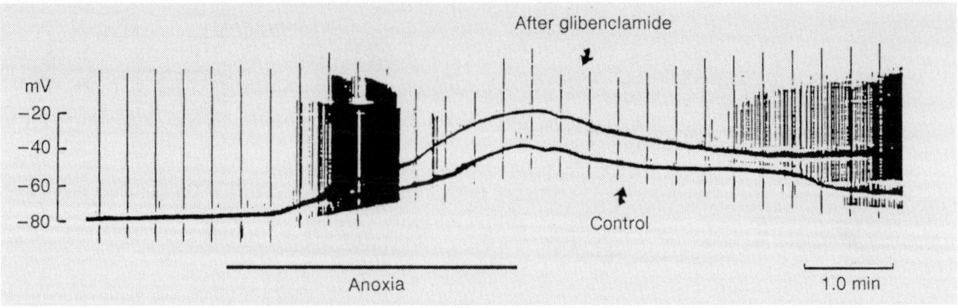

Fig. 2. Intracellular recordings before, during and after anoxia in an adult hypoglossal neuron before and after use of glibenclamide, a specific blocker of ATP-sensitive K^+ channels. Note that the depolarization is more prolonged and exaggerated with glibenclamide than with control [J Neurophysiol 1991;66:103–111].

importance in the response and adaptation of central neurons [3, 6, 19]. Activation of K_{ATP} channels on postsynaptic membranes of hypoglossal neurons tends to hyperpolarize or limit the depolarization of these neurons in conditions that can lower intracellular ATP levels [19] (fig. 2). The importance of these K_{ATP} channels therefore stems from their role in reducing membrane excitability during anoxia and hence in decreasing energy consumption and preserving cytosolic high-energy phosphates. In the hippocampus, anoxia-induced activation of K_{ATP} channels, presumed to be on the presynaptic membrane of CA3 neurons, hyperpolarizes presynaptic terminals, decreases excitatory neurotransmitter release and leads to hyperpolarization of pyramidal neurons [3]. Hyperpolarization would reduce energy consumption and prevent activation of several cation channels, reduce energy expenditure and have a protective effect when central neurons are exposed to O_2 deprivation.

Other Potential Channel Mechanisms

Although K_{ATP} channels may be involved in mediating loss of intracellular K^+, other mechanisms can be as important [25–28]. For example, an increase in excitability and action potential generation in neurons will induce an increased leakage of K^+ [2, 4, 25, 26]. Similarly, since Ca_i^{2+} increases in some neurons (hippocampal), Ca^{2+}-activated K^+ channels would be another mechanism [2, 25, 26]. It would be interesting also to speculate that Na^+-activated K^+ channels may play a role during anoxia since Na_i^+ is most likely increased to levels that would influence the gating of this channel [6].

As indicated in the introductory statements, we believe that K^+ channels are not the only ones that play an important role during anoxia [6, 27]. Indeed, there are intricate interactions between mitochondrial, membrane, cytosolic and nuclear events during anoxia with a number of channels being involved [6]. One of our major findings recently had to do with the role and importance of Na^+ channels and transport during O_2 deprivation [27]. We have recently shown, for example, that voltage-sensitive Na^+ currents are inhibited in a major way in adult central neurons [27]. This inhibition was mostly due to the left-shift in the steady state inactivation kinetics of the Na^+ channel (and therefore to the decrease in the activatable number of Na^+ channels) during anoxia. Interestingly, this was not seen in newborn central neurons but in those of the adult [27]. The mechanism(s) underlying this difference is not well understood at this stage.

Acknowledgements

This work was supported by NIH grants HL 39924 and HD 15736 and 28940. C. Jiang is a Fellow of the Parker Francis Family Foundation.

References

1 Choi DW: Ionic dependence of glutamate neurotoxicity in cortical cell culture. J Neurosci 1987;7:369–379.
2 Krnjević K, Leblond J: Changes in membrane currents of hippocampal neurons evoked by brief anoxia. J Neurophysiol 1989;62:15–30.
3 Ben Ari Y, Krnjević K, Crepel V: Activators of ATP-sensitive K^+ channels reduce anoxic depolarization in CA3 hippocampal neurons. Neuroscience 1990;37:55–60.
4 Haddad GG, Donnelly DF: O_2 deprivation induces a major depolarization in brain stem neurons in the adult but not in the neonatal rat. J Physiol 1990;429:411–428.
5 Donnelly DF, Jiang C, Haddad GG: Comparative responses of brainstem and hippocampal neurons to O_2 deprivation: In vitro intracellular studies. Am J Physiol 1992;262: L549–554.
6 Haddad GG, Jiang C: O_2 deprivation in the central nervous system: On mechanisms of neuronal response, differential sensitivity and injury. Prog Neurobiol 1993;40: 277–318.
7 Stick TJ, Rosenthal M, LaManna JC, Lutz PL: Brain potassium ion homeostasis, anoxia, and metabolic inhibition in turtles and rats. Am J Physiol 1982;243:R281–288.
8 Stick TJ, Chasnoff EP, Rosenthal M: Potassium ion homeostasis and mitochondrial redox status of turtle brain during and after ischemia. Am J Physiol 1985;248:R531–R540.
9 Chih CP, Feng ZC, Rosenthal M, Lutz PL, Sick TJ: Energy metabolism, ion homeostasis, and evoked potentials in anoxic turtle brain. Am J Physiol 1989;257:R854–R860.
10 Chih CP, Rosenthal M, Sick TJ: Ion leakage is reduced during anoxia in turtle brain: A potential survival strategy. Am J Physiol 1989;257: R1562–1564.
11 Haddad GG, Donnelly DF: Tolerance to anoxia in newborm mammals and reptiles: Intracellular neuronal studies. Soc Neurosci Abstr 1989;15:1194.
12 Siesjö BK: Historical overview: Calcium, ischemia, and death of brain cells. Ann NY Acad Sci 1988;522: 638–661.
13 Choi DW: Cerebral hypoxia: Some new approaches and unanswered questions. J Neurosci 1990;10: 2493–2501.
14 Ashcroft FM: Adenosine 5′-triphosphate-sensitive potassium channels. Annu Rev Neurosci 1988;11:97–118.
15 Ashford MLJ, Sturgess NC, Trout NJ, Gardner NJ, Hales CN: Adenosine-5-triphosphate-sensitive ion channels in neonatal rat cultured central neurons. Pflügers Arch 1988; 412:297–304.
16 Ashford MLJ, Boden PR, Treherne JM: Glucose-induced excitation of hypothalamic neurons is mediated by ATP-sensitive K^+ channels. Pflügers Arch 1990;415:479–483.
17 Hansen AJ: Extracellular potassium concentration in juvenile and adult rat brain cortex during anoxia. Acta Physiol Scand 1977;99:412–420.
18 Hansen AJ: The extracellular potassium concentration in brain cortex following ischemia in hypo- and hyperglycemic rats. Acta Physiol Scand 1978;102:324–329.
19 Jiang C, Haddad GG: Effect of anoxia on intracellular and extracellular potassium activity in hypoglossal neurons in vitro. J Neurophysiol 1991;66:103–111.
20 Jiang C, Xia Y, Haddad GG: Role of ATP-sensitive K^+ channels during anoxia: Major differences between rat (newborn, adult) and turtle neurons. J Physiol (Lond) 1992; 448:599–612.
21 Xia Y, Haddad GG: Major differences in CNS sulfonylurea receptor distribution between rat (newborn, adult) and turtle. J Comp Neurol 1991;314:278–289.
22 Norma A: ATP-regulated K^+ channels in cardiac muscle. Nature 1983; 305:147–148.
23 Schmid-Antomarchi H, Amoroso S, Fosset M, Lazdunski M: K^+ channel openers activate brain sulfonylurea-sensitive K^+ channels and block neurosecretion. Proc Natl Acad Sci USA 1990;87:3489–3492.
24 Davies NW: Modulation of ATP-sensitive K^+ channels in skeletal muscle by intracellular protons. Nature 1990;343:374–377.
25 Krnjević K, Cherubini E, Ben-Ari Y: Anoxia on slow inward currents of immature hippocampal neurons. J Neurophysiol 1989;62:896–906.
26 Leblond J, Krnjević K: Hypoxic changes in hippocampal neurons. J Neurophysiol 1989;62:1–14.
27 Cummins TR, Donnelly DF, Haddad GG: Effect of oxygen deprivation on the excitability of isolated hippocampal CA1 neurons: Developmental aspects. J Neurophysiol 1991;66:1471–1482.
28 Xia Y, Jiang C, Haddad GG: Oxidative and glycolytic pathways in rat (newborn, adult) and turtle brain: Role during anoxia. Am J Physiol 1992;262:R595–603.

Biol Neonate 1994;65:166–170

M.P. Morin-Surun[a]
E. Boudinot[a]
T. Schäfer[b]
M. Denavit-Saubié[a]

[a] Institut Alfred-Fessard, Biologie Fonctionnelle du Neurone, CNRS, Gif-sur-Yvette, France;
[b] Abteilung für Angewandte Physiologie, Ruhr-Universität, Bochum, BRD

Brain Stem Chemosensitivity: Its Implication in Central Respiratory Regulation

Key Words
Isolated adult brain stem
Chemoreceptors
Extracellular fluid
Cerebrospinal fluid
Hypercapnia
In vitro
Guinea pig

Abstract
Central brain stem chemosensitivity plays an essential role in acid-base regulation. The site of the chemosensitive neuronal elements has not yet been clearly established. To address this question, we used an in vitro adult guinea pig isolated brain stem preparation, maintained in survival conditions by intra-basilar and bath perfusions of Krebs solution saturated with 95% O_2 and 5% CO_2. Hypercapnic stimulation, produced by modifying the CO_2 concentration of the medium perfusing brain stem structures via the basilar perfusion system, increased the respiratory burst frequency recorded from the hypoglossal nerve. Hypercapnia evoked by ventral surface superfusion increased the respiratory burst amplitude. These data suggest that chemosensitive neuronal elements could be located at the ventral surface as well as in the deeper brainstem structures. However, their characteristics may be different.

Introduction

After the discovery of the carotid and aortic glomera, investigators began to consider peripheral and central chemoreceptors as separate entities. Evidence that the ventrolateral aspects of the medulla oblongata (VLM) might be involved in the central pH/pCO_2-sensitive mechanism was first reported by Loeschke's group (1958, see [1]), perfusing the cerebral ventricles with mock CSF of varied pH at constant pCO_2 and vice versa.

Different chemosensitive areas have been defined by Schlaefke et al. (1970, see [1]). They used a concentric double superfusion probe to differentiate pH-sensitive areas 1 mm^2-wise and cold block, and described three areas [1–3]. Bilateral cool block of the

M.P Morin-Surun, MD
Institut Alfred-Fessard
Equipe de Biologie Fonctionnelle du Neurone
CNRS
F–91198 Gif-sur-Yvette Cedex (France)

0006–3126/94/
0654–0166$5.00/0

intermediate area causes apnea when aortic and sinus nerves are cut. This effect leads to the working hypothesis that the information from both chemosensitive fields (rostral and caudal areas) would converge within the intermediate area, from where it would be relayed to the respiratory integrative network. Evidence for central chemosensitive areas on the ventral medullary surface of other species has been also demonstrated (rat [4]; dog [5]) but so far nothing definitive is known about the H^+ ion sensitivity characteristics of the ventral brain stem surface of man. However, histopathological findings on the ventral medullary surface of sudden infant death victims provide some hints that this area may play a vital role in man as well [1].

Several attempts have been made to record neurons within the chemosensitive sites of the VLM that are implicated in the chemoreception process. Some correlations have been found among the firing rates of cells, the acidity of the VLM and the ventilatory pattern [6, 7]. However, there is no evidence that these different responses were not evoked by synaptic events. Recently, Takeda and Haji [8] have shown that respiratory neurons located in the ventral respiratory area (nucleus ambiguus) had a synaptic response to hypercapnic stimulation. On the other hand, in brain slices, neurons of the nucleus tractus solitarius demonstrate a membrane potential depolarization when submitted to a hypercapnic medium [9]. This depolarization persists after synaptic blockade, indicating a direct effect on the neuronal membrane.

This result re-emphasizes the question about the location of the central chemoreceptors. It is possible that neurons mediating this response are spread throughout the brain stem. To dissociate the actions of hypercapnia on brain stem structures from those on the ventral brain stem surface, we used the in vitro adult guinea pig brain stem preparation, maintained in survival conditions by intrabasilar and bath perfusions of the Krebs solution saturated with 95% O_2 and 5% CO_2. For this question, our preparation presents several advantages: (1) the functional respiratory network is preserved and isolated from peripheral and rostral afferents [10]; (2) we can establish the ionic composition and the CO_2 concentration of both perfused and superfused Krebs solutions; (3) we can independently control the 'extracellular fluid' (ECF) by the perfusion through the basilar artery and the 'cerebrospinal fluid' (CSF) by the bath superfusion. We have shown that if all the brain stem structures could participate in the respiratory response to hypercapnic stimulation, their respiratory responses can be dissociated.

Material and Methods

Data were obtained from 7 adult guinea pigs (200–320 g) anesthetized with sodium pentobarbital (30 mg/kg i.p.), decapitated at the first cervical vertebra and decerebrated at the intercollicular level. The brain stem (with the cerebellum) was rapidly removed from the cranium. During this surgical procedure, cold (4 °C) Krebs solution was dripped onto the exposed brain surfaces. The brain stem was secured by fine pins with the ventral surface orientated upwards, in a recording chamber filled with Krebs at room temperature. The basilar artery was cannulated rapidly with a catheter inserted at the level of the pons, and the vascular system was perfused with Krebs at room temperature using a Gilson pump (1.6–2 ml/min). Ends of arteries at the cervical first segment of the spinal cord were ligated. The pia was completely removed from the ventral surface. The entire surface of the brain stem was completely immersed and continuously superfused at a constant rate (2–2.5 ml/min) in the chamber (fig. 1). The Krebs solution consisted of (in m*M*): NaCl 124, KCl 5, $MgSO_4$ 2.2, KH_2PO_4 1.2, $NaHCO_3$ 26, $CaCl_2$ 2, glucose 10 and was saturated with 95% O_2 and 5% CO_2 (pH 7.38 ± 0.06 SEM). Respiratory activity was monitored from hypoglossal roots through a glass suction electrode. Nerve activity was amplified and filtered with a Grass model P5 preamplifier. Half-

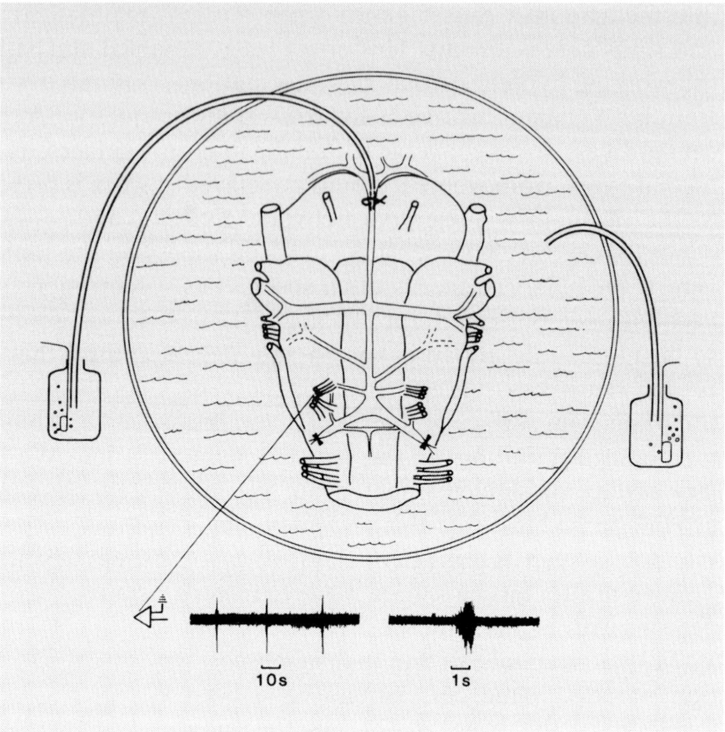

Fig. 1. Schematic representation of the in vitro brain stem preparation of an adult guinea pig. The brain stem is exposed with the ventral surface facing up. Superficial vascularisation and nerve roots are drawn. Recording of the respiratory activity of the hypoglossal roots is presented below the preparation.

wave activity of hypoglossal roots was integrated through a passive RC integrating circuit (time constant 20 ms). All signals were displayed on an oscilloscope and recorded on digital tape and displayed on a thermal recorder (Ankersmit).

Hypercapnic acidic Krebs was obtained by increasing the fractional concentration of CO_2 bubbling (to 10.9% ± 1.67 SEM) the Krebs solution ($NaHCO_3$ 26 m*M*) to achieving pH 7.01 (± 0.07 SEM). CO_2 concentration bubbling the solution was measured with an infrared CO_2 gas analyzer (Cosma). Test solutions were perfused through the basilar artery for 3 min and superfused into the bath for at least 15 min. These times ensured equilibration of the respective solutions.

The periodic activity recorded from hypoglossal roots consisted of a burst of activity corresponding to inspiration followed by low-amplitude tonic expiratory activity. The amplitude of the inspiratory burst was determined from the integrated form of the hypoglossal neurogram.

Results

Figure 2 illustrates the pattern of the inspiratory activity recorded from the hypoglossal nerve submitted to hypercapnic acidic Krebs superfused onto the ventral surface (bath application) followed by a hypercapnic acidic perfusion into the brain stem structures (basilar perfusion).

Respiratory Effects Induced by Changes of the CO_2 Partial Pressure and pH through the Bath

The hypercapnic acidic medium (pH 7.07 ± 0.03 SEM, CO_2 10.4% ± 0.7 SEM, n = 5) superfused via the bath increased the inspiratory burst amplitude within the 10 min of application (9.9 min ± 1.3 SEM, n = 5). This duration corresponds to the time required to

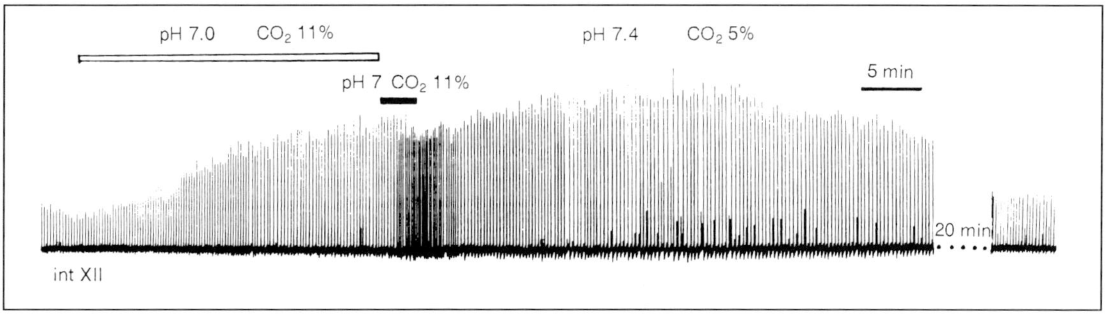

Fig. 2. Differential effects of hypercapnic acidic medium injected on the ventral surface by the bath perfusion (white bar) and in the brain stem structures by the basilar perfusion (black bar). Int XII = Integration of the inspiratory activity of the hypoglossal nerve.

equilibrate the bath. In most cases, this effect was followed by an increase in the respiratory burst frequency during the recovery.

Respiratory Effects Induced by Changes of the CO_2 Partial Pressure and pH through the Basilar Artery

When the control medium was replaced (for 3 min) by a hypercapnic acidic medium (pH 7.0 ±0.06 SEM, CO_2 11.3% ±0.6 SEM, n = 7), the respiratory burst frequency increased. In most cases (n = 5/7), this increase was associated with a decrease in the burst amplitude. Recovery was attained within 7.1 min (± 1 min).

Discussion

The main finding from this study is that the surface as well as deeper brain stem structures are implicated in the response to a hypercapnic acidic perfusion. However, the type of respiratory response is different according to the areas affected.

Many studies have reported an increase in the respiratory amplitude following a hypercapnic acidic perfusate applied to the ventral surface as we have also described in this study [1, 2]. However, nobody has described the increase in the respiratory burst frequency that we observed after intrabasilar perfusion of an hypercapnic acidic medium. In vivo, intravertebral artery injection of CO_2-saturated saline evoked a simultaneous increase in both respiratory parameters associated with an acidic shift of ECF pH [11]. Since a high density of small arterioles and venules are located close to the ventral surface [12], the hypercapnic acidic medium may be not only transported over the brainstem but also interact with neurons located at the ventral surface. In our experiments, this effect on the ventral surface could be diminished since the bath perfusion maintained the ventral surface in normal Krebs during the basilar hypercapnic acidic injection.

In the in vitro newborn rat brain stem preparation maintained in survival conditions by a bath perfusion, central respiratory chemosensitivity has also been demonstrated [13, 14]. In vitro study of the central respiratory-like activity of the fetal rat has demonstrated that the fetal respiratory-like activity appears at day 16 and stabilises at day 20 when it becomes sensitive to CO_2 and pH stimuli [15]. Central chemosensitivity maturation is thus closely related to the respiratory brain stem maturation. However, there is an age difference in the responsiveness of brain stem chemosensitive neurons to extracellular pH changes [16]. A loss of central chemosensitivity could be a cause of the 'sudden infant death syndrome' (SIDS) [1] and a better understanding of chemosensitivity mechanisms and their maturation could provide a new therapeutic approach for the predisposed SIDS infants.

Acknowledgments

This work was supported by CNRS and by a grant from DRET 92.075. Dr T. Schäfer has an ENP Short-Term Fellowship.

References

1 Schlaefke ME: Central chemosensitivity: A respiratory drive. Rev Physiol Biochem Pharmacol 1981;90:171–244.

2 Loeschke HH: Central chemosensitivity and the reaction theory. J Physiol (Lond) 1982;332:1–24.

3 Millhorn DE, Eldridge L: Role of the ventrolateral medulla in the regulation of respiratory and cardiovascular systems. J Appl Physiol 1986;61:1249–1263.

4 Tojima H, Kuriyama T, Fukuda Y: Differential respiratory effects of HCO_3 and CO_2 applied on the ventral medullary surface of the rats. J Appl Physiol 1991;70:2217–2225.

5 Chonan T, Adams EM, von Euler C, Cherniack NS: Effects of focal cooling in the ventrolateral medulla on chemoresponsiveness in dogs. Respir Physiol 1990;80:45–54.

6 Trouth CO, Patrickson JW, Holloday JA, Wright LE: Neurophysiological studies on superficial medullary chemosensitive area for respiration. Brain Res 1982;246:47–56.

7 Arita H, Ichikawa K, Kuwana S, Kogo N: Possible locations of pH-dependent central chemoreceptors: intramedullary regions with acidic shift of extracellular fluid pH during hypercapnia. Brain Res 1989;485:285–293.

8 Takeda R, Haji A: Synaptic response of bulbar respiratory neurons to hypercapnic stimulation in peripherally chemodenervated cats. Brain Res 1991;561:307–317.

9 Dean JB, Bayliss DA, Erickson JT, Lawing WL, Millhorn DE: Depolarization and stimulation of neurons in nucleus tractus solitarii by carbon dioxide does not require chemical synaptic input. Neuroscience 1990;36:207–216.

10 Morin-Surun MP, Boudinot E, Sarraseca H, Fortin G, Denavit-Saubié M: Respiratory network remains functional in a mature guinea pig brainstem isolated in vitro. Exp Brain Res 1992;90:375–383.

11 Ichikawa K, Kuwana S, Arita H: ECF pH dynamics within the ventrolateral medulla: A microelectrode study. J Appl Physiol 1989;67:193–198.

12 Cragg P, Patterson L, Purves MJ: The pH of the brain extracellular fluid in the cat. J Physiol (Lond) 1977;272:137–166.

13 Harada Y, Kuno M, Wang YZ: Differential effects of carbon dioxide and pH on central chemoreceptors in the rat in vitro. J Physiol (Lond) 1985;368:679–693.

14 Monteau R, Morin D, Hilaire G: Acetylcholine and central chemosensitivity: In vitro study in the newborn rat. Respir Physiol 1990;81:241–254.

15 Di Pasquale E, Monteau R, Hilaire G: In vitro study of the central respiratory-like activity of the fetal rat. Exp Brain Res 1992;89:459–464.

16 Whittaker JAC, Trouth CO, Pan Y, Millis RM, Bernard DG: Age differences in responsiveness of brainstem chemosensitive neurons to extracellular pH changes. Life Sci 1990;46:1699–1705.

Biol Neonate 1994;65:171–175

M. Denavit-Saubié[a]
M. Kalia[b]
O. Pierrefiche[a]
P. Schweitzer[a]
A.S. Foutz[a]
J. Champagnat[a]

[a] Institut Alfred-Fessard, Equipe de Biologie Fonctionnelle du Neurone, CNRS, Gif-sur-Yvette, France;
[b] Department of Neurosurgery, Thomas Jefferson University, Philadelphia, Pa., USA

Maturation of Brain Stem Neurons Involved in Respiratory Rhythmogenesis: Biochemical, Bioelectrical and Morphological Properties

Key Words
Maturation
Respiratory
Nucleus tractus solitarius
I_A current
Glutamate
Neuronal morphology
NMDA

Abstract
Neonatal and adult respiratory-related functions of brain stem were compared using in vivo or in vitro approaches. The control of inspiratory off-switch by glutamate-like neurotransmitters was found active at birth. However, neurons from the nucleus tractus solitarius (NTS) are immature at birth because they present growth cones and the transient potassium current appears progressively during the first week of life in association with modification of the dendritic tree. These data support the hypothesis that the mechanisms of respiratory rhythmogenesis are different at birth and in the adult.

Introduction

The neuronal network which generates respiration is spontaneously active throughout life and eleborates a periodic pattern of discharge which can be easily recognized. This neuronal network is located in the brain stem at the level of the obex [1, 2] and includes the nucleus tractus solitarius (NTS) which receives input from pulmonary chemoreceptors and baroreceptors via the vagus and glossopharyngeal nerves and modulates automatic rhythmic activities. Motor respiratory output depends on the integration of properties of the neuronal network such as intrinsic bioelectric function, morphology, pattern of interconnectivity and specificity of neuronal responses to different putative neurotransmitters. In order

M. Denavit-Saubié
Institut Alfred-Fessard
Equipe de Biologie Fonctionnelle du Neurone
CNRS
F–91198 Gif-sur-Yvette Cedex (France)

0006–3126/94/
0654–0171$5.00/0

to elucidate the role played by development in the system, the interrelationship of maturation with each one of these functional properties must be examined.

An important mechanism in respiratory rhythmogenesis is the 'off switch' which is responsible for the abrupt passage from inspiration to expiration, and involves vagal input as well as brain stem microcircuitry. In the absence of vagal feedback, glutamate activation of NMDA (N-methyl-*D*-aspartate) receptors is essential to produce off-switch in adults [3]. In neonate, brain stem respiratory mechanisms differ considerably from the adult [4–6]. Consequently, it is of interest to test whether NMDA receptors are already involved in early life.

Brain stem muturation processes are also important at the elementary level because elaboration of rhythmic activity depends on neuronal bioelectric properties [7, 8]. A typical feature of adult NTS neurons is the large amplitude and duration of transient outward currents [9–11]. One component of these outward currents is referred as I_A currents which occur when the neuronal membrane potential passes from a hyperpolarisation phase to a depolarisation. This I_A current whose amplitude is particularly high in the adult solitary complex [9, 10] induces inhibition. During the first week of postnatal life, synaptic properties of NTS neurons indicate an increased excitability of these cells as compared with their adult counterparts [12, 13]. This could be the consequence of a reduction of I_A currents and should be tested in neonates.

Other developmental processes occur in the morphology of neurons in the brain stem respiratory network. Early studies using the Golgi technique [14] suggested that the NTS neurons undergo rapid and dramatic changes in morphology during postnatal development [15]. The timing of these morphological changes may correlate closely with the timing of some electrophysiological modification of neurons recorded in brain stem slices [12, 13].

Experimental Technique

In vivo studies were performed on newborn kittens aged 6 h to 2 days and adult cats. Respiratory activity was measured with the barometric method. Blockade of NMDA receptors was obtained by intravenous administration of the NMDA antagonist MK 801 [16]. Bilateral vagotomy was performed under halothane anesthesia.

In vitro studies were performed on brain stem slices [9, 10]. NTS neurons were recorded either after intracellular impalement or in the whole-cell patch clamp configuration, the usual microelectrode solution being (in m*M*): NaCl (10); K gluconate (125); Hepes (10); EGTA (11); $CaCl_2$; $MgCl_2$ (2); Mg ATP (2,5), glucose (10); pH 7.28. Biocytin was dissolved in this microelectrode solution in a concentration of 0.5%, in order to label the recorded cells for further study of their morphology.

Results

Comparison of the Effect of NMDA Receptor Blockade in Kitten and in Adult Cat

In the control state, the kittens had a rapid and variable breathing pattern with expirations (TE) longer than inspirations (TI). After intraperitoneal injection of 6 mg/kg of MK 801, kittens lay motionless with a more regular breathing pattern and a clear increase of the duration of inspiration which in some cases led to apneusis (long inspiratory pauses). As a consequence of the reduced respiratory frequency, minute volume was substantially depressed although tidal volume was not modified (fig. 1).

After bivagotomy (fig. 1), apneusis was observed in all kittens (n = 7). Mean TI was increased 4-fold while TE remained stable. The results obtained in kittens by blockade of

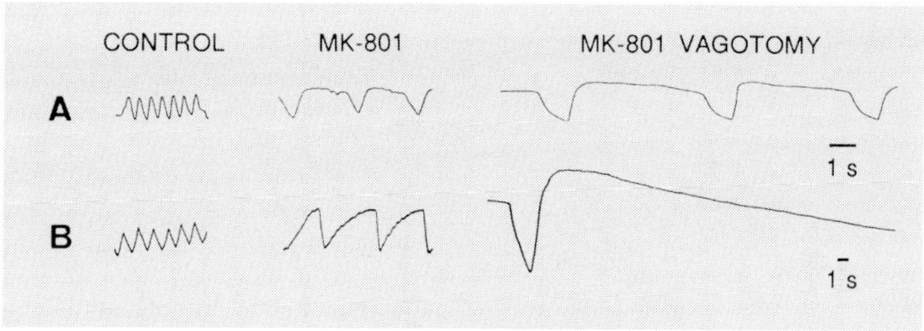

Fig. 1. Comparison between effect of MK-801 administration on the breathing pattern of newborn (**A**) and adult (**B**) cats before (middle) and after vagotomy (right). Inspiration is upward.

NMDA receptors are comparable to those obtained in bivagotomized adult cats, but in adults apneusis was obtained with smaller doses of MK 801 (1 mg/kg). We conclude from these results that blockade of NMDA receptors causes similar effects in adult and newborn.

Comparison of IA Current in Adult and Newborn Cat

In vitro brain stem slices are better adapted that in vivo experiments to the current clamp and voltage clamp measurements of nucleus tractus solitarius (NTS) neurons. In adult, measurements of most NTS neurons present a transient inactivating outward current which was revealed by depolarization to –30 to –45 mV after a conditioning hyperpolarization to potentials of –60 to –100 mV. Amplitude of this outward current was particularly important in NTS neurons as compared with other brain neurons. This IA current which is recorded with a high probability in adult NTS was much less frequent in newborn NTS neurons. A study performed on 108 NTS neurons in animals between postnatal days 0–9, demonstrates that during this period the number of cells which presented this transient inhibitory I_A current increased progressively. Fifty percent or neurons showed I_A in days P3 to P9 as compared with days P0 to P2. These results reveal the dynamic nature of neurons in the NTS during early development.

Comparison of Morphology in Mature and Immature NTS Neurons Based on the Presence of I_A Current

Slices containing the recorded NTS neurons filled with biocytin were processed to determine their location and morphology. Electrophysiological and morphological data were collected and analyzed in a double-blind manner. Data comparison showed that morphologics of I_A positive NTS neurons are remarkably different from I_A-negative cells (fig. 2). I_A-positive neurons recorded in adult or during the late developmental phase have a multipolar (bushy) appearance while I_A-negative neurons recorded during the early developmental phase had bipolar dendritic trees (polarized in two opposite directions).

Discussion

The present results show that the maturation process is different according to the functional properties of the respiratory networks. While some neurotransmitter mechanisms (such as those involving NMDA receptors) are mature at birth, other processes related to morphological and bioelectrical properties are still immature.

The effect of MK 801 alone and in association with vagotomy is qualitatively similar in kittens and in adult cats [3] and adult monkey [17]. Thus, the central NMDA receptor-me-

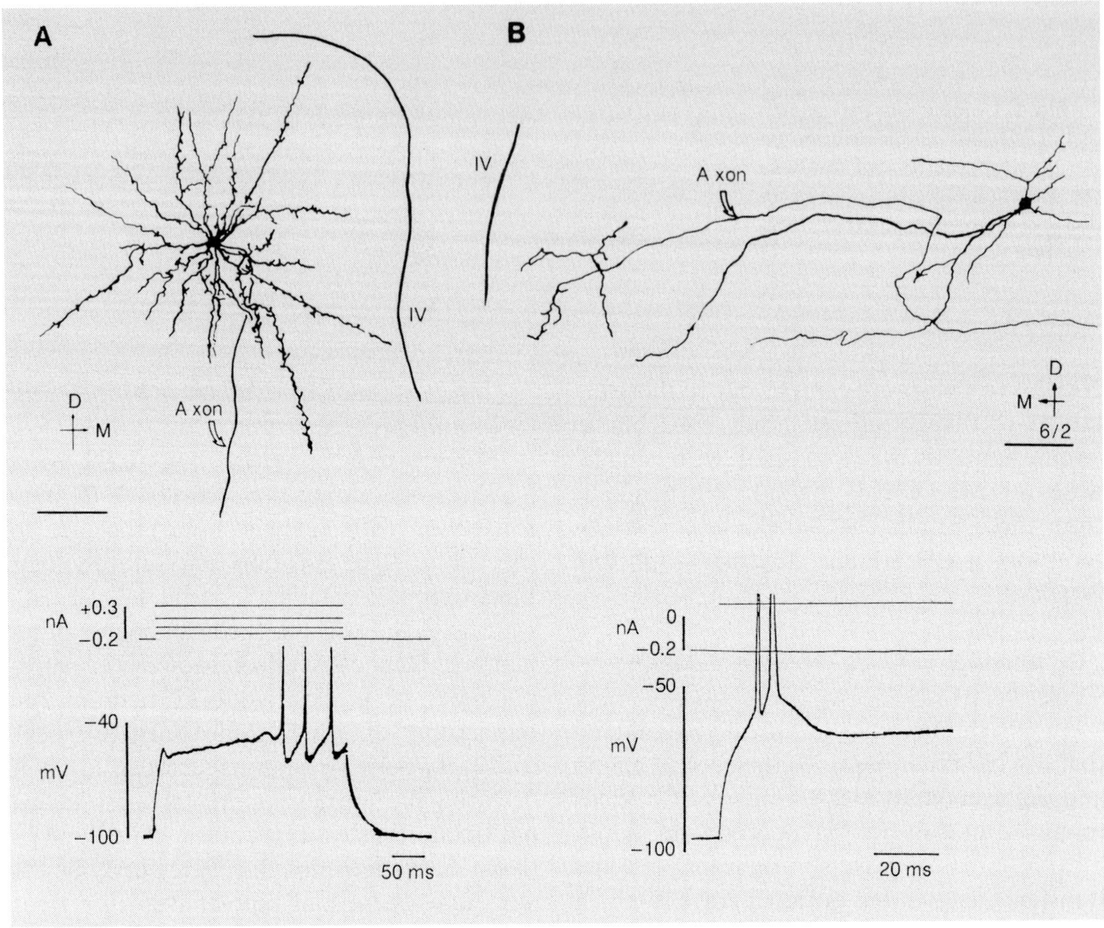

Fig. 2. Comparison between morphological and bioelectrical properties of adult-like I_A positive (**A**) and immature I_A negative (**B**) neurons of the nucleus tractus solitarius.

diated 'off switching' mechanism is already functional in the first days of postnatal life.

In contrast to this maturity of NMDA receptors at birth, the bioelectric properties of NTS neurons are still immature. The electrophysiological maturation closely matches with morphological differentiation. This morphogenesis includes an increase in the complexity of the dendritic tree from a bipolar to a multipolar appearance. It has been proposed that the number of afferents terminating on a neuron determines the size and complexity of its dendritic trees [18]. It may be hypothetized that the shape of the dendritic tree is secondary to the maturation of vagal afferents in the rat during the first postnatal week.

Acknowledgement

This work was supported by the CNRS, Fondation pour la Recherche Médicale and Fondation Naître et Vivre.

References

1 Bianchi AL: Localisation et étude des neurones respiratoires bulbaires. Mise en jeu antidromique par stimulation spinale ou vagale. J Physiol (Paris) 1971;63:5–40.

2 Cohen MI: Neurogenesis of respiratory rhythm in the mammal. Physiol Rev 1979;59:1105–1173.

3 Foutz AS, Champagnat J, Denavit-Saubié M: Involvement of N-methyl-*D*-aspartate (NMDA) receptors in respiratory rhythmogenesis. Brain Res 1989;500:199–208.

4 Marlot D, Duron B: Postnatal development of vagal control of breathing in the kitten. J Physiol (Paris) 1979; 75:891–900.

5 Schweitzer P, Pierrefiche O, Foutz AS, Denavit-Saubié M: Effects of N-methyl-*D*-aspartate (NMDA) receptor blockade on breathing pattern in newborn cat. Dev Brain Res 1990; 56:290–293.

6 Trippenbach T: Developmental aspects of respiratory reflexes; in Euler C von, Lagercrantz H (eds): Neurobiol Control Breathing. New York, Raven Press, 1986, pp 283–290.

7 Takashima S, Becker LE: Prenatal and postnatal maturation of medullary respiratory centers. Dev Brain Res 1986;26:173–177.

8 Quattrochi JJ, McBride PT, Yates AJ: Brain stem immaturity in sudden death syndrome: A quantitative rapid Golgi study of dendritic spines in 95 infants. Brain Res 1985;325: 39–48.

9 Champagnat J, Denavit-Saubié M, Grant K, Shen KF: Organization of synaptic transmission in the mammalian solitary complex, studied in vitro. J Physiol 1986;381:551–573.

10 Champagnat J, Jacquin T, Richter DW: Voltage-dependent currents in neurones of the solitary tract of rat brain stem slices. Pflügers Arch 1986;406:372–379.

11 Dekin MS, Johnson S, Getting PA: In vitro characterization of neurons in the ventral part of the nucleus tractus solitarius in guinea pigs. Identification of neuronal types and repetitive firing properties. J Neurophysiol 1987;58:195–214.

12 Haddad GG, Getting PA: Repetitive firing properties of neurons in the ventral region of nucleus tractus solitarius. In vitro studies in adult and neonatal rat. J Neurophysiol 1989;62:1213–1224.

13 Schweitzer P, Fortin G, Beloeil JC, Champagnat J: In vitro study of newborn rat brain maturation: Implication of sudden infant death syndrome. Neurochem Int 1992;20: 109–112.

14 Cajal RY: Histologie du système nerveux de l'homme et des vertébrés. Reprinted by Instituto Ramon y Cajal del CSIC 1952.

15 Kalia M: Early ontogeny of the vagus nerve: An analysis of the medulla oblongata and cervical spinal cord of the postnatal rat. Neurochem Int 1992;20:119–128.

16 Wong EHF, Kemp JA, Priestley T, Knight AR, Woodruff GN, Iversen LL: The anticonvulsant MK-801 is a potent N-methyl-*D*-aspartate antagonist. Proc Natl Acad Sci USA 1986; 83:7104–7108.

17 Pierrefiche O, Foutz AS, Denavit-Saubié M: Pneumotaxic mechanisms in the non-human primate: Effect of the N-methyl-*D*-aspartate (NMDA) antagonist ketamine. Neurosci Lett 1990;119:90–93.

18 Leventhal AG, Schall JD, Ault SJ: Extrinsic determinants of retinal ganglion cell development in the cat. J Neurosci 1988;8:2028–2038.

Biol Neonate 1994;65: 176–181

D. Morin
E. Di Pasquale
G. Hilaire
R. Monteau

Biologie des Rythmes et du Développement, URA 205, Faculté St-Jérôme, Marseille, France

Possible Involvement of Serotonin in Obstructive Apnea of the Newborn

Key Words
Serotonin
Respiration
Obstructive apnea
Newborn

Abstract
Experiments were conducted on newborn rats in order to study the serotonergic modulation of the central respiratory activity during the neonatal period. In vitro experiments performed on isolated brainstem spinal cord preparations demonstrated that serotonin exerts a permanent excitatory modulation on the central respiratory rhythm generator but depresses the inspiratory motor output to the genioglossus muscle. In vivo experiments confirmed that increasing endogenous serotonin levels decreases the inspiratory activity of the genioglossus and elicits drastic obstructive apneas.

In this paper, we summarize previous reports on the postnatal modulation of central respiratory activity exerted by serotonin (5-HT). Some of these results were obtained on the in vitro brain stem-spinal cord of the neonatal rat, in which rhythmic inspiratory discharges can still be recorded from the cervical and cranial respiratory nerves [1]. Briefly, 5-HT has been found to modulate both the frequency and the motor output of the respiratory centers, and in particular to depress the activity of the hypoglossal (XII) nerve. Since the EMG activity of the genioglossus muscle (GG, innervated by the XII) has been reported to either decrease or completeley disappear during obstructive apnea (OA), the 5-HT-induced depression of the XII motor output might be relevant to OA. As our results were obtained using a reduced in vitro preparation it seemed to be necessary to test this hypothesis using more classical in vivo models, i.e. freely breathing anesthetized newborn rats: these experiments confirmed that activation of 5-HT biosynthesis depresses the GG activity and induces drastic OA. These findings are discussed in the light of clinical data which suggest that OA and abnormal central 5-HT levels might occur in cases of sudden infant death syndrome (SIDS).

Prof. R. Monteau
Biologie des Rythmes et du Développement
URA 0205
Faculté St-Jérôme
F-13397 Marseille Cedex (France)

0006–3126/94/
0654–0176 $5.00/0

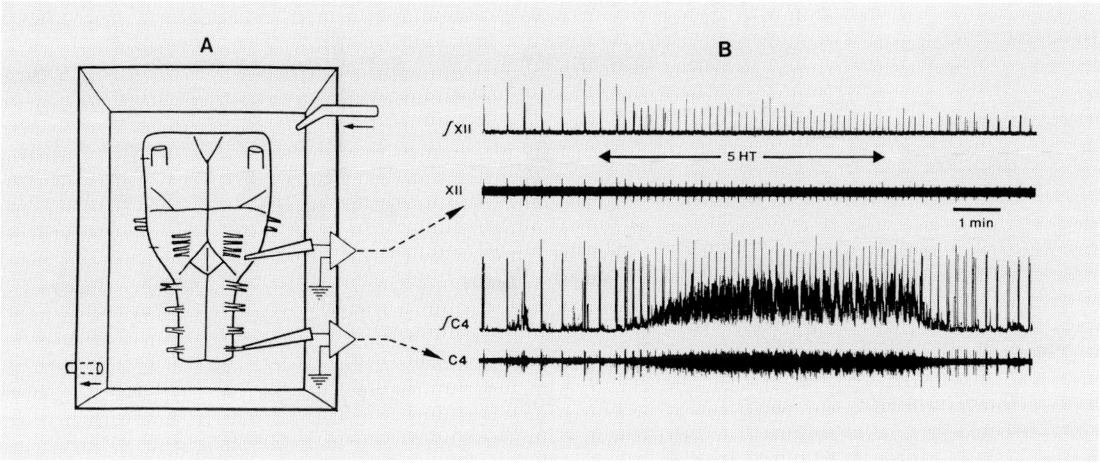

Fig. 1. In vitro effects of medium containing 5-HT (30 μ*M*) on the amplitude of the inspiratory discharge of XII nerve and cervical ventral root. **A** Schematic drawing of the ventral surface of the preparation in the recording chamber and the recording electrodes. **B** From top to bottom, integrated and raw discharges of the XII nerve and cervical ventral root under normal medium and under 5-HT (between arrows). Note (i) the increase in respiratory frequency; (ii) the tonic discharge and the persistence of the respiratory rhythm in the cervical recording; (iii) the decrease in XII amplitude.

In vitro Experiments

In vitro experiments were performed on 0- to 3-day-old newborn rats, which were anesthetized with ether and then decerebrated. The brain stem and spinal cord placed in a chamber filled with artificial cerebrospinal solution warmed at 27 ± 0.5 °C and equilibrated with 95% O_2 and 5% CO_2, continued to produce respiratory discharges [1] which were recorded from the cervical ventral roots and/or the XII nerve (suction electrodes, fig. 1A) and from motoneurons (intracellular micropipettes).

Effects of 5-HT on the Central Respiratory Activity of the Brain Stem-Spinal Cord Preparation

The effects of replacing the normal medium by a medium containing 5-HT (30 μ*M*) were of 3 types (fig. 1): a 5-HT_1 increase in respiratory frequency, a 5-HT_2 tonic activation in the cervical roots and a 5-HT_2 depression of the inspiratory XII discharge.

5-HT_1 Excitatory Modulation of Respiratory Frequency. 5-HT was found to increase the respiratory frequency by 50% within 1–2 min and by using specific 5-HT agonists and antagonists it was observed that this effect was mediated by 5-HT_1 sites [2] in the rostral ventrolateral medulla [3]. Applying drugs known to interact with 5-HT mechanisms affected the respiratory frequency: 5-HT uptake inhibitor (fluoxetine, 100 μ*M*) and 5-HT precursors (*L*-tryptophan, 50 μ*M*; 5-hydroxytryptophan, 50 μ*M*) increased the respiratory rate by 33, 42 and 56%, respectively, while 5-HT antagonist (methysergide, 50 μ*M*) decreased the respiratory frequency by 15%. These experiments demonstrate that: (i) 5-HT biosynthesis mechanisms remain functional in vitro, and (ii) a continuous 5-HT release exerts an

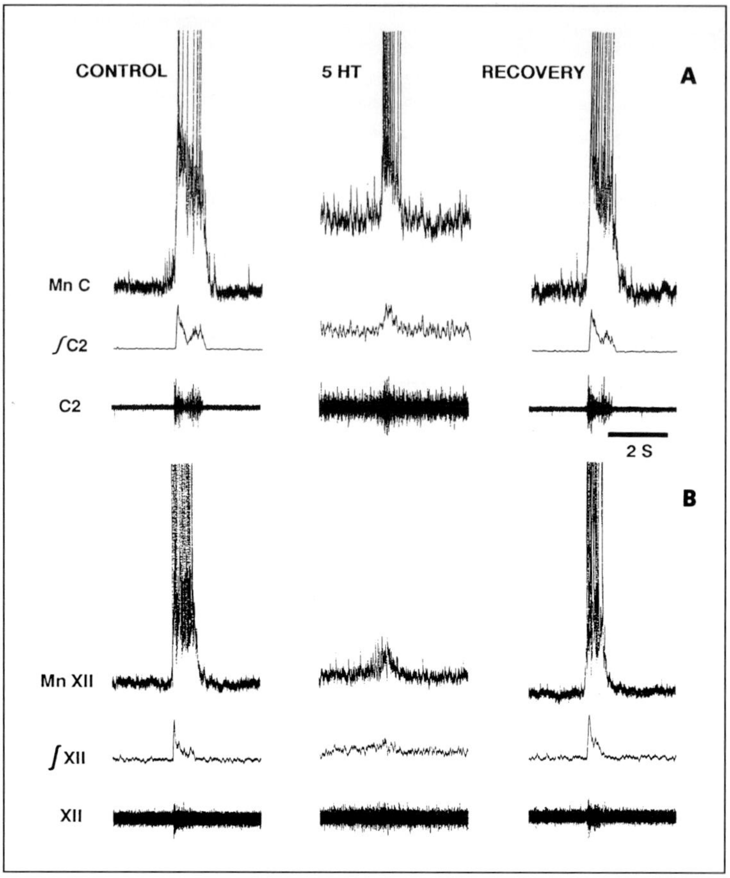

Fig. 2. In vitro effects of 5-HT on the intracellularly recorded activity of both inspiratory cervical and hypoglossal motoneurons. **A** Cervical motoneuron. **B** XII motoneuron; in each panel the tracings correspond to the intracellular recording and the integrated and raw discharge of the corresponding nerve. Note (i) the phasic inspiratory depolarization in both motoneurons during both control and recovery; (ii) the persistence of this drive superimposed on a strong depolarization at the cervical level, as compared with its reduction to a subthreshold level and the absence of depolarization in the XII motoneuron.

excitatory modulation on the respiratory rhythm generator via medullary 5-HT_1 sites.

5-HT_2 Facilitation of Cervical Motor Output. Under 5-HT medium, a tonic discharge occurred on the cervical ventral roots, superimposed on the respiratory bursts; this tonic firing involved spinal 5-HT_2 receptors and was mainly due to the recruitment of previously silent nonrespiratory motoneurons, while the inspiratory ones generally continued to produce phasic inspiratory firing although they occasionally delivered a few spikes during expiration [4].

5-HT_2 Depression of XII Motor Output. Applying media containing 5-HT agents (5-HT, 5-HT precursors, specific agonists and antagonists) and activating the raphe nuclei depressed, or completely suppressed, the inspiratory activity of the XII nerve by activating 5-HT_2 receptors [2, 5–7]. Since local application of 5-HT restricted to the XII nucleus also depressed the XII discharge [8], it was assumed that the depression was due to a local 5-HT action within the XII nucleus.

Intracellular Analysis of the 5-HT_2 Depression of XII Motoneurons

On brain stem-spinal cord preparation, 5-HT-induced changes were analyzed intracellularly (fig. 2) [4, 8]. Cervical inspiratory motoneurons were activated because 5-HT (i) induced a large depolarization of the

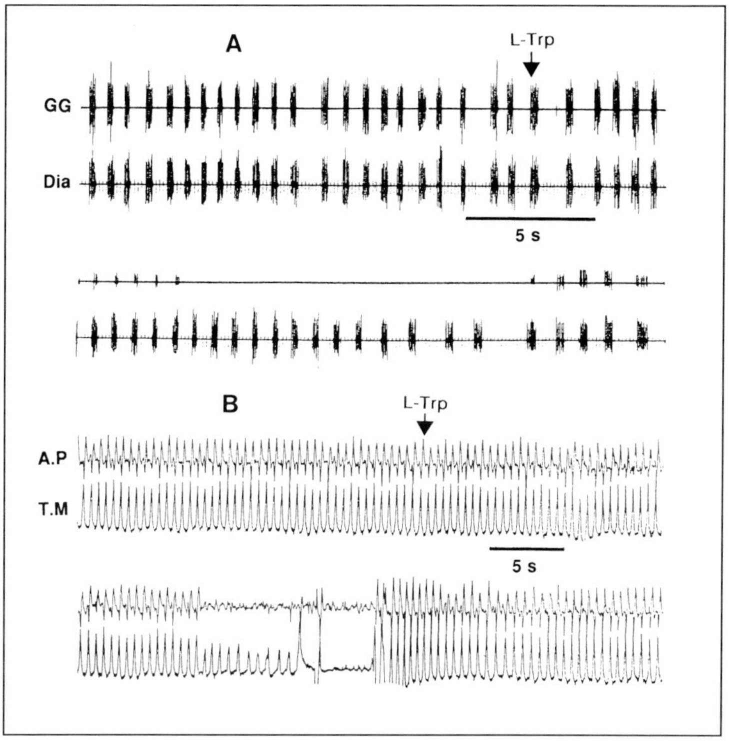

Fig. 3. In vivo effects of i.p. injection of *L*-trp. **A, B** injection of *L*-trp (arrow). **A** EMG activity of GG and diaphragm (Dia) under control conditions and 25 min after *L*-trp. Note that GG activity decreased and even disappeared but not that of the diaphragm. **B** Upper airway pressure changes (upper trace) and chest movements (lower trace, inspiration upward) under control conditions (top) and 25 min after *L*-trp. Note the occurrence of episodes of OA followed by central apnea.

membrane potential; (ii) increased the input membrane resistance, and (iii) did not affect the amplitude of the central inspiratory drive. Conversely, XII motoneurons were silenced because 5-HT (i) induced only a slight depolarization; (ii) did not affect the input membrane resistance, and (iii) decreased the amplitude of the central inspiratory drive.

In vivo Experiments

Anesthetized (pentobarbital, i.p. <10 mg·kg^{-1}) freely breathing newborn rats (3–10 days) received i.p. injection of *L*-tryptophan (*L*-trp, 50 mg/kg).

Induced Changes in 5-HT Biosynthesis

In 68 newborn rats (10 litters), the cerebrospinal fluid levels of 5-HT and 5-HIAA were analyzed by HPLC prior to and after *L*-trp. Large individual variations were noted even between rats from the same litter, of the same age and weight, but the 5-HT levels increased significantly (Mann-Whitney nonparametric test) within 30 min of the injection whereas the 5-HIAA levels were increased but not significantly.

5-HT-Induced Depression of the XII Motor Output

In 26 newborn rats (7 litters), the EMG activity of the diaphragm and that of the GG was recorded prior to and after *L*-trp. The amplitude of the GG discharge dropped to 40% of the control level within 30 min of the *L*-trp injection, while the diaphragmatic firing was not significantly affected. The GG discharge occasionally stopped completely for a few successive breaths (fig. 3A) or for a few minutes. These effects could be prevented by applying a pretreatment at birth with PCPA (300 mg·kg^{-1}), which blocked the 5-HT biosynthesis from *L*-trp.

5-HT-Induced Obstructive Apnea (OA)

In newborn rats (13 litters), the chest respiratory movements and the resulting airway pressure changes were monitored both prior to and after *L*-trp injection. In 7 litters, most of the newborn rats (21/25) displayed OA within 20–40 min of the *L*-trp injection (fig. 3B). These disorders recurred frequently (every 5–6 min), became longer (10–30 s) and were followed by central apnea lasting for several seconds. Recovery was generally achieved within 45–60 min, but in 2 newborn rats, episodes of OA and central apnea occurred, which worsened until death. No OA were ever observed after i.p. injections of (i) saline (n = 5); (ii) *L*-trp after 5-HT antagonist pretreatment (methysergide i.p. 50 mg·kg^{-1}, n = 5), and (iii) *L*-trp after PCPA pre-treatment (n = 7).

In 6 other litters, *L*-trp did not elicit any respiratory disorders among the 18 newborn rats tested, which had the same age and weight as those which displayed OA; no obvious particularity was detected which might explain their insensitivity to *L*-trp.

The results of in vitro experiments showed that 5-HT depresses the XII inspiratory discharge by activating 5-HT$_2$ receptors located within the hypoglossal nucleus. This depression might be due to a presynaptic action on the axon terminals arising from the respiratory centers impinging on the XII motoneurons. Our in vivo results confirmed this hypothesis, since increases in central 5-HT levels depressed the GG activity and elicited drastic OA in half of the newborn rats.

Central respiratory disorders are commonly suspected in SIDS [9] but the results of the numerous SIDS studies which have been carried out in the respiratory field have often been contradictory: sleep apneas have often been reported [10] but so have normal pneumograms [11]. The finding that 5-HT biosynthesis activation elicits drastic, and even lethal, OA in the newborn rat might be of great significance as regards SIDS, since these victims have been reported to show (i) signs of hypoxemia and intrathoracic petechiae which might result from OA [9]; (ii) abnormal histological profiles on central respiratory neurons [12, 13] as well as on GG motoneurons [12], and (iii) abnormally high levels of the 5-HT metabolite, 5-HIAA, which suggest that an increase in the 5-HT biosynthesis levels occurs prior to death [14]. The 5-HT mechanisms are not yet fully mature at birth, and considerable changes in the 5-HT, 5-HIAA [15], and 5-HT2 receptor mRNA levels [16] occur postnatally. The processes regulating these developmental changes are still unknown, but it can be speculated that any disturbances (in utero suffering, environmental and nutritional changes, etc.) which might affect the maturation of the 5-HT mechanism at a particular developmental stage might result in respiratory and other vegetative disorders. In the future, defining why *L*-trp elicits OA in some newborn rats but not in others should constitute a major step towards understanding SIDS, but whether the results obtained on newborn rats can be extrapolated to newborn infants still remains an open question.

Acknowledgements

This research was supported by the CNRS, the INSERM, the Ministère de la Santé, the Conseil Régional PACA and the 'Naître et Vivre' Foundation.

References

1 Hilaire G, Monteau R, Errchidi S: Possible modulation of the medullary rhythm generator by the noradrenergic A5 area: An in vitro study in the newborn rat. Brain Res 1989; 485:325–332.

2 Morin D, Hennequin S, Monteau R, Hilaire G: Serotonergic influences on central respiratory activity: An in vitro study in the newborn rat. Brain Res 1990;535:281–287.

3 Di Pasquale E, Morin D, Monteau G, Hilaire G: Serotonergic modulation of the respiratory rhythm generator at birth: An in vitro study in the rat. Neurosci Lett 1992;143:91–95.

4 Morin D, Monteau R, Hilaire G: Serotonin and cervical respiratory motoneurons: Intracellular study in the newborn rat brainstem-spinal cord preparation. Exp Brain Res 1991;84:229–232.

5 Monteau R, Morin D, Hennequin S, Hilaire G: Differential effects of serotonin on respiratory activity of hypoglossal and cervical motoneurons: An in vitro study on the newborn rat. Neurosci Lett 1990;111:127–132.

6 Morin D, Hennequin S, Monteau R, Hilaire G: Depressant effect of raphe stimulation on inspiratory activity of the hypoglossal nerve: In vitro study in the newborn rat. Neurosci Lett 1990;116:299–303.

7 Morin D, Monteau R, Hilaire G: 5-HT modulates central respiratory activity of the newborn rat: in vitro study. Eur J Pharmacol 1991;192: 89–95.

8 Morin D, Monteau R, Hilaire G: Compared effect of 5-HT on the inspiratory activity of hypoglossal and cervical motoneurons: An in vitro study in the newborn rat. J Physiol (Lond) 1992;451:605–630.

9 Kinney H, Filiano J, Harper R: The neuropathology of the Sudden Infant Death Syndrome. A review. J Neuropathol Exp Neurol 1992;51: 115–126.

10 Schechtman V, Harper R, Wilson A, Southall D: Sleep apnoea in infants who succumb to the sudden infant death syndrome. Pediatrics 1991; 87:841–846.

11 Rahilly PM: Pneumographic studies: Predictors of future apnoeas but not sudden infant death in asymptotic infants. Aust Paediatr J 1989; 25:211–214.

12 Quattrochi J, McBride P, Yates A: Brainstem immaturity in Sudden Infant Death Syndrome: A quantitative rapid Golgi study of dendritic spines in 95 infants. Brain Res 1985; 325:39–48.

13 Takashima S, Becker LE: Developmental abnormalities of medullary 'respiratory centers' in sudden infant death syndrome. Exp Neurol 1985;90:580–587.

14 Caroff J, Girin E, Alix D; Cann-Moisan C, Sizun J, Barthélémy L: Neurotransmission et mort subite du nourrisson. Etude du liquide céphalo-rachidien. C R Acad Sci Paris 1992;314:451–454.

15 Hamon M, Bourgoin S: Characteristics of 5-HT metabolism and function in the developing brain; in Osborne NN (ed): Biology of Serotonergic Transmission. New York, Wiley, 1982, pp 197-220.

16 Roth B, Hamblin M, Ciaranello R: Developmental regulation of 5-HT2 and 5-HT1C mRNA and receptor levels. Dev Brain Res 1991;58:51–58.

Biol Neonate 1994;65:182–188

Carlos E. Blanco

Department of Neonatology,
University of Limburg,
Maastricht, The Netherlands

Maturation of Fetal Breathing Activity

Key Words
Fetal breathing movement
Fetal lambs

Abstract
Spontaneous breathing movements are present during fetal life and they are important for normal development of the lung. Early in gestation they seem to represent free-running activity of the respiratory centers, not controlled by peripheral mechanisms but probably dependent on a tonic CO_2 drive. Maturation of sleep states brings into play powerful brainstem inhibitory mechanisms which control FBM. At birth these mechanisms must be overridden to allow the establishment of continuous breathing.

Fetal breathing movements (FBM) are present in utero from early in gestation despite an environment almost free of stimuli. They seem to be under very little reflex control [1, 2]. They are very irregular in frequency and amplitude in early gestation, reflecting spontaneous activity of central structures in the brain stem. In this situation most, if not all, of the classical stimuli which regulate and control breathing activity are not present, or if present they seem to be below threshold.

FBM represent brain stem output since they are associated with phrenic and diaphragmatic activity and they produce small tidal movements of tracheal fluid [3, 4]. The first evidence of some type of regulation becomes evident with the differentiation of the electroencephalographic activity (ECoG) and behavioral states as described in animals [2, 5, 6]. The lack of peripheral control is suggested by several experiments; vagotomy [2, 7–12] or chemoreceptor denervation does not modify the incidence of breathing activity.

Origin and Control of Spontaneous Fetal Breathing Movements During Pregnancy

FBM are present in fetuses of many species including man [13, 14]. Since breathing activity is not responsible for providing gas exchange, this raises the question of the function

Carlos E. Blanco MD
Department of Neonatology
University of Limburg
NL–6200 MD Maastricht (The Netherlands)

0006–3126/94/
0654–0182 $5.00/0

of such oxygen-consuming fetal activity [15]. Several studies show a direct correlation between lung growth and the presence of FBM, by either decreasing [16, 17] or increasing its incidence [18] or by increasing the fetal thoracic wall compliance and therefore diminishing the intrathoracic pressure generated by FBM [19]. Thus, it is clear that FBM play an important role in fetal lung growth and development.

Sleep States

Early in gestation in animals [20, 21] and man [5, 14, 22] breathing activity is present almost continuously and is associated with increased activity in the postural muscles of the neck and limbs [21]. At the same time the ECoG activity is undifferentiated (low amplitude, frequencies of around 10 Hz). This is different from the low voltage during REM sleep seen after differentiation. During the last trimester of pregnancy in the sheep, breathing activity becomes clearly associated with, or limited by, maturation of the ECoG or behavioral states. The ECoG differentiates into alternating episodes of high voltage, low frequency (3–10 Hz; HVECoG) and low voltage, high frequency (17–35 Hz; LVECoG) activity, frequently termed quiet and REM sleep. Breathing activity begins to be clearly episodic just before maturation of the ECoG; at this time FBM are associated with rapid eye movements, increased activity of the nuchal muscles [21] and an increased amplitude of polysynaptic spinal reflexes [23]. After differentiation breathing activity becomes organized into a distinctive pattern; it is present during LVECoG and associated with rapid eye movements, absence of nuchal muscle activity, and inhibition of polysynaptic spinal reflexes [24]; and is inhibited during periods of HVECoG. Therefore, it is clear that with ECoG differentiation two new states start to play a role in the modulation of breathing in utero. It is present in periods of variable duration for 30–40% of the total time or 60–70% of LVECoG time, is very irregular in amplitude and in frequency. This variability demands long periods of observation when planning experiments in order to avoid results due to chance.

Mechanism for Lack of FBM during HVECoG

Little is known about the mechanisms which cause inhibition of FBM during HVECoG and how they are switched off during LVECoG. Transection at the level of the inferior colliculus, although not at the level of the optic chiasm, cause FBM to become dissociated from ECoG and eventually to become continuous. This suggests that apnea during HVECoG may result from active inhibition originating from midbrain or the upper pons [25]. Periodic inhibition of FBM apparently involves the midbrain or the upper pons, the coordination of FBM and ECoG depending on the integrity of pathways between this area and the cortex. Gluckman and Johnston [26, 27] produced small bilateral lesions in the lateral pons and observed a dissociation of FBM from ECoG, breathing during HVECoG (but not continuous breathing) and stimulation of FBM during hypoxia. Furthermore, fetal lactic acidosis or hypercapnia caused continuous FBM only in fetuses with lesions and not in intact fetuses. They concluded that the absence of FBM during HVECoG is the consequence of a raised threshold and a descending inhibitory process which involves the rostral lateral pons. This area seems to be involved in both inhibition of breathing during GVECoG and during hypoxia.

A lack of peripheral input has been suggested to be one of the mechanisms involved in the fetal apnoea during HVECoG. This is supported by experiments where regular FBM (even during HVECoG) and shivering were induced by the stimulation of cutaneous thermoreceptors [28]. The effect on FBM may, however, be mediated by the increase in metabolism consequent upon cooling. By using ECMO in chronic preparations we observed stimulation of FBM when fetal central temperature fell by 2 °C, but this effect decreased or disappeared during hypocapnia [Kuipers and Blanco, unpubl. observations]. This suggests that an increased production of CO_2 plays an important role in the response.

Several drugs have been reported to overcome the apnoea during HVECoG, i.e. serotonin precursors 5-HTP [29], *L*-5-HTP [30], inhibitors of prostaglandin synthesis [31], pilocarpine [32, 33], morphine [34], thyrotropin-releasing hormone [35, 36]. These studies are promising but much more research is needed to clarify the mechanisms involved in the regulation of spontaneous breathing.

After cord occlusion at birth the inhibition of breathing activity during HVECoG must be overridden and breathing must become continuous. Several simultaneous changes are present at birth which can be responsible for lifting the inhibition of breathing seen during HVECoG in utero. The disappearance of an inhibitory substance of placental origin has been recently proposed as a possible mechanism for the establishment of continuous breathing at birth [37]. We could not confirm this hypothesis when using ECMO to support the fetus and control blood gases during cord occlusion in fetal lambs [38].

Carbon Dioxide

The role of CO_2 is highlighted by observations where newborn lambs presented spontaneous breathing while on artificial ventilation only during REM sleep provided that they were normocapnic. However, breathing activity disappeared when these lambs were hypocapnic [39]. During fetal hypocapnia, induced by maternal hyperventilation in human [40] and animals [41], breathing activity decreased or disappeared. This supports the view that the level of CO_2 is an important drive for the generation of breathing activity in utero. Recently, we used an extracorporeal system (ECMO) in chronically instrumented lambs to produce fetal hypocapnia directly. Under these circumstances breathing activity was barely present or absent for period of up to 6 hours, reappearing as soon as the CO_2 level was increased to baseline levels [Kuipers and Blanco, unpubl. observations]. Thus, CO_2 is an important drive for the respiratory centers (central chemoreceptor) in the fetus and it seems to determine the presence of breathing activity during LVECoG in utero. However, despite a continuous CO_2 drive or even under hypercapnic conditions, breathing is not present during HVECoG suggesting an active inhibition or a decrease in CO_2 sensitivity of the central chemoreceptor during this state. Evidence for central inhibitory mechanisms in combination with raised threshold of the central chemoreceptor was provided by observations made in fetal lambs with bilateral lesions rostral to the trigeminal nuclei and at the level of the Vth nerve and middle cerebellar peduncle [27]. In those lambs breathing activity was absent during HVECoG in normocapnia but it became almost continuous during hypercapnia through both states and dissociated from eye movements and nuchal muscle activity.

What determines the presence of breathing activity early in gestation is not known, but the respiratory pattern-generating mechanisms may begin to function spontaneously and independent of afferent input as in isolated neonatal brain stem preparations [42, 43]. Later in gestation FBM are limited to LVECoG and dependent on the level of CO_2 [Kuipers and Blanco, unpubl. observations]. Therefore, it could be hypothesized that early in gestation FBM are present because the central generators of breathing become sensitive to CO_2.

Hypercapnia

Hypercapnia causes stimulation of fetal breathing movements in animals and man after birth. Fetal hypercapnia produced by maternal inhalation of 4–6% CO_2 in air or by using ECMO, increases the incidence of FBM, its depth and the inspiratory slope and FBM become more regular [7, 44–46]. However, this response is limited to LVECoG; HVECoG is still inhibitory regardless of the level of PCO_2. This response has been described in fetal lambs from 75 days [47]. In the human the response is present after the 24th week of gestation and its sensitivity increases as gestation advances [42]. Peripheral chemoreceptor denervation does not change the response [11]. However, lesions in the lateral pons 'allowed' the presence of FBM in HVECoG during hypercapnia [27]. Therefore, central chemoreception is present in fetal life and apnea during HVECoG is due to a decrease in its sensitivity. Although this response is similar to that seen after birth, it is not logical in fetal life since the increase in 'fetal ventilation' will not correct fetal PCO_2 and fetal oxygen consumption will increase. The existence of this illogical response could support the idea that CO_2 drive is essential for the presence of FBM and underline its importance as a crucial mechanism for the establishment of breathing at birth.

Oxygenation

Oxygen delivery in utero, despite the 'hypoxemic' PaO_2 (25–30 mm Hg) values compared to after birth, is adequate since it matches oxygen consumption and it allows for fetal activity and growth. However, recent reports [48] suggest that fetal PaO_2, despite normal oxygen availability, might be sensed as hypoxia by central mechanisms. This could trigger tonic inhibition which might contribute to the absence of FBM during HVECoG. In order to test this hypothesis techniques like mechanical ventilation, ECMO or hyperbaric maternal oxygenation have been used to increase fetal PaO_2 in chronically instrumented fetal lambs. Baier et al. [48] reported an association between the occurrence of continuous FBM and fetal PaO_2 levels >200 mm Hg. This PaO_2 could have markedly reduced fetal cerebral blood flow making the interpretation of these results difficult [49]. However, when fetal PaO_2 was increased to neonatal levels using hyperbaric maternal oxygenation this association was not observed [50]. By using ECMO in chronically instrumented fetal lambs we increased fetal PaO_2 to levels between 60 and 90 mm Hg and kept fetal PCO_2 at control levels for periods up to 19 h. In this situation, we did not observe any change in the incidence of FBM [51].

The role of PaO_2, in the initiation of breathing activity after cord clamping is less clear, since at birth PaO_2 is physiologically low and only increases when breathing activity is already initiated. However, once breathing is initiated oxygenation is crucial for its maintenance.

Response to Hypoxia

In contrast to after brith, acute decrease in oxygen availability to the tissues obtained either by decreasing oxygen content (reducing PaO_2 or hemoglobin [7, 52, 43]) or by histotoxic hypoxia (oligomycin [54]) triggers central inhibitory mechanism resulting in inhibition of FBM, body movements, muscle activity, spinal reflexes, and causes a switching to a higher voltage and more synchronized ECoG rather than producing arousal [7, 21, 55, 56]. These inhibitory mechanisms are dependent on gestational age since inhibition is less pronounced earlier than 115 days in the fetal sheep. It is interesting to note that at this time in gestation FBM begin to be inhibited during HVECoG, which could suggest common mechanisms acting during hypoxia and HVECoG. The lack of stimulation of breathing and arousal during hypoxia is not due to the absence of chemoreceptor function since they are functional and responsive in utero [57]. Direct depression of the medullary respiratory centers is not the cause either, since hypoxia causes stimulation of FBM after suprapontine brain stem transection [25] or placement of lesions [26] or reversible cooling of small areas in the lateral pons [58].

These observations suggest either that the increased activity of the chemoreceptors in hypoxia is insufficient to elicit a respiratory response or that hypoxia activates inhibitory mechanisms within the brainstem which make the respiratory centers insensitive to this afferent input. Evidence for the latter can be found in experiments using unanesthetized fetal lambs where the carotid and aortic chemoreceptor were denervated and either the brainstem was transected [12, 59] or the lateral pons was lesioned [13, 26, 27]. In these experiments brain stem transection or lesions in the pons 'permitted' a respiratory response during fetal hypoxia. However, after subsequent carotid chemoreceptor denervation this response disappeared and the incidence of FBM decreased during normoxia. This indicates again that peripheral chemoreceptor can exert a tonic stimulatory respiratory drive but in the intact animals this activity remains subthreshold for the brain stem. Recent neurophysiological studies in newborn lambs identified areas within the pons, more medial but close to the area described by Gluckman and Johnston [26], in which some neurons showed an increase in their discharge during hypoxia. Electrical stimulation of these areas produced apnea [60]. Therefore, these pontine areas are involved in the inhibition of FBM either as chemoreceptor by sensing oxygen availability or by mediating and integrating the inhibitory process. Utilization of drugs with hypoxiamimetic actions, like almitrine, might clarify this point in the future [61]. The role of adenosine in this inhibitory process has been proposed [59]. Since the methods used to induce fetal hypoxia are maternal hypoxia or reducing uterine flow, a blood-borne chemical factor produced elsewhere might be involved in the response. However, FBM and fetal states were not influenced during maternal hypoxemia when fetal PaO_2 was kept at normoxic or even mild hyperoxic by using ECMO in utero [62]. This indicates that the inhibition during hypoxia originated within fetal tissues and is triggered by a decrease in oxygen availability. What happens to these mechanism after birth is not clear, but there are situations resembling fetal responses during the neonatal period, e.g. apnea or periodic breathing. It is clear that at birth the inhibitory mechanisms triggered by HVECoG and hypoxia are overridden to allow continuous breathing. It is also clear that peripheral chemoreceptors reset their sensitivities to the new range of neonatal values. This could avoid PO_2 values dropping to near the values which triggered the inhibitory response in utero.

In conclusion, spontaneous breathing movements are present during fetal life and they are important for normal development of the lung. Early in gestation they seem to represent free-running activity of the respiratory centers, not controlled by peripheral mechanisms but probably dependent on a tonic CO_2 drive. Maturation of sleep states brings into play powerful brain stem inhibitory mechanisms which control FBM. At birth these mechanisms must be overridden to allow the establishment of continuous breathing.

References

1 Barcroft J, Barron DH: The genesis of respiratory movements in the fetus of the sheep. J Physiol 1937;88: 56–61.

2 Dawes GS, Fox HE, Leduc BM, Liggins GC, Richards RT: Respiratory movements and rapid eye movements sleep in the foetal lamb. J Physiol 1972;220:119–143.

3 Bahoric A, Chernick V: Electrical activity of phrenic nerve and diaphragm in utero. J Appl Physiol 1975;39:513–518.

4 Maloney JE, Adamson TM, Brodecky V, Cranage S, Lambert TF, Ritchie BC: Diaphragmatic activity and lung liquid flow in the unanesthetized fetal sheep. J Appl Physiol 1975;39:423–428.

5 Patrick J, Champbell K, Carmichael L, Natale R, Richardson B: Patterns of human fetal breathing during the last 10 weeks of pregnancy. Obstet Gynecol 1980;56:24–30.

6 Trudinger BJ, Knight PC: Fetal age and patterns of human fetal breathing movements. Am J Obstet Gynecol 1980;137:724–728.

7 Boddy K, Dawes GS, fisher R, Pinter S, Robinson JS: Foetal respiratory movements, electrocortical and cardiovascular responses to hypoxemia and hypercapnia in sheep. J Physiol 1974;243:599–618.

8 Condorelli S, Scarpelli EM: Fetal breathing: Induction in utero and effects of vagotomy and barbiturates. J Pediatr 1976;88:94–101.

9 Jansen AH, Ioffe S, Russell BJ, Chernick V: Effect of carotid chemoreceptor denervation on breathing in utero and after birth. J Appl Physiol 1981;51:630–633.

10 Rigatto H, Hasan SU, Jansen A, Gibson D, Nowaczyk B: The effects of total peripheral denervation on fetal breathing and on the establishment of breathing at birth in sheep; in Jones CT (ed): Fetal and Neonatal Development. Ithaca, Perinatology Press, 1988, pp 613–621.

11 Koos BJ, Sameshima H: Effects of hypoxaemia and hypercapnia on breathing movements and sleep state in sinoaortic-denervated fetal sheep. J Dev Physiol;10:131–144.

12 Moore PJ, Parkes MJ, Nijhuis JG, Hanson MA: The incidence of breathing movements of fetal sheep in normoxia and hypoxia after peripheral chemodenervation and brain-stem transection. J Dev Physiol 1989;11:147–151.

13 Johnston BM: Brain stem inhibitory mechanisms in the control of fetal breathing movements; in Hanson MA (ed): The Fetal and Neonatal Brain Stem: Developmental and Clinical Issues. Cambridge, University Press, 1991, pp 21–47.

14 Boddy K, Dawes GS: Fetal breathing. Br Med Bull 1975;31:3–7.

15 Rurak DW, Grubner NC: Increased oxygen consumption associated with breathing activity in fetal lambs. J Appl Physiol 1983;54:701–707.

16 Wigglesworth JS, Desai R: Effects on lung growth of cervical cord section in the rabbit fetus. Early Hum Dev 1979;3:51–65.

17 Liggins GC, Vilos GA, Campos GA, Kitterman JA, Lee CH: The effects of spinal cord transection on lung development in fetal sheep. J Dev Physiol 1981;3:267–274.

18 Nagai A, Thurlbeck WM, DeBoeck C, Ioffe S, Chernick V: The effects of maternal CO_2 breathing on lung development of their fetuses: Morphology and morphometric studies. Am Rev Respir Dis 1987;135:130–136.

19 Liggins GC, Vilos GA, Campos GA, Kitterman JA, Lee CH: The effect of bilateral thoracoplasty on lung development in fetal sheep. J Dev Physiol 1981;3:275–282.

20 Bowes G, Adamson TM, Ritchie BC, Dowling M, Wilkinson MH, Maloney JE: Development of patterns of respiratory activity in unanesthetized fetal sheep in utero. J Appl Physiol 1981;50:693–700.

21 Clewlow F, Dawes GS, Johnston BM, Walker DW: Changes in breathing, electrocortical and muscle activity in unanesthetized fetal lambs with age. J Physiol 1983;341: 463–476.

22 Natale R, Nasello-Paterson C, Connors G: Patterns of fetal breathing activity in humans fetus at 24 to 28 weeks of gestation. Am J Obstet Gynecol 1988;158:317–321.

23 Rigatto H, Blanco CE, Walker DW: The response to stimulation of hindlimb nerves in fetal sheep, in utero, during the different phases of electrocortical activity. J Dev Physiol 1982;4:175–185.

24 Blanco CE, Dawes GS, Walker DW: Effects of hypoxia on polysynaptic hindlimb reflexes of unanesthetized fetal and newborn lambs. J Physiol 1983;339:453–466.

25 Dawes GS, Gardner WN, Johnston BM, Walker DW: Breathing in fetal lambs: The effects of brain stem section. J Physiol 1983;335:535–553.

26 Gluckman PD, Johnston BM: Lesion in the upper lateral pons abolish the hypoxic depression of breathing in unanesthetized fetal lambs in utero. J Physiol 1987;382: 373–383.

27 Johnston BM, Gluckman PD: Lateral pontine lesions affect central chemosensitivity in unanesthetized fetal lambs. J Appl Physiol 1989;67: 1113–1118.

28 Gluckman PD, Gunn TR, Johnston BM: The effects of cooling on breathing and shivering in unanesthetized fetal lambs in utero. J Physiol (Lond) 1983;343:395–506.

29 Quilligan E, Clewlow F, Johnston B, Walker D: Effects of 5-hydroxytryptophan on electrocortical activity and breathing movements of fetal sheep. J Obstet Gynecol 1981;141: 271–275.

30 Fletcher DJ, Hanson MA, Moore PJ, Nijhuis JG, Parkes MJ: Stimulation of breathing movements by L-5-Hydroxytryptophan in fetal sheep during normoxia and hypoxia. J Physiol 1988;404:575–589.

31 Kitterman JA, Liggins GC, Clements JA, Tooley WH: Stimulation of breathing movements in fetal lambs by inhibitors of prostaglandin synthesis. J Dev Physiol 1979;1: 453–466.

32 Brown ER, Lawson EE, Jansen A, Chernick V, Taeusch HW: Regular fetal breathing induced by pilocarpine infusion in the near-term fetal lamb. J Appl Physiol 1981;50:1348–1352.

33 Hanson MA, Moore PJ, Nijhuis JG, Parkes MJ: Effects of pilocarpine on breathing movements in normal, chemodenervated and brain stem-transected fetal sheep. J Physiol 1988;400:415–424.
34 Hasan SU, Lee D, Gibson DA, Nowaczyk BJ, Cates DB, Sitar DS, Pinsky C, Rigatto H: Effects of morphine on breathing and behavior in fetal sheep. J Appl Physiol 1988;64: 2058–2065.
35 Umans JG, Umans HR, Szeto HH: Effects of thyrotropin-releasing hormone in the fetal lamb. Am J Obstet Gynecol 1986;155:1266–1271.
36 Bennet L, Gluckman PD, Johnston BM: The central effects of thyrotropin releasing hormone on the breathing movements and electrocortical activity of the fetal sheep. Pediatr Res 1988;23:72–75.
37 Adamson SL, Kuipers IM, Olson DM: Umbilical cord occlusion stimulates breathing independent of blood gases and pH. J Appl Physiol 1991;70:1796–1809.
38 Kuipers IM, Maertzdorf WJ, Keunen H, De Jong DS, Hanson MA, Blanco CE: Fetal breathing is not initiated after cord occlusion in the unanaesthetized fetal lamb in utero. J Dev Physiol 1992;17:233–240.
39 Henderson-Smart DJ, Johnson P, McLelland ME: The abolition of spontaneous breathing during quiet sleep by eupneic positive pressure ventilation in lambs. J Physiol 1980; 307:48P–49P.
40 Connors G, Hunse C, Carmichael L, Natale R, Richardson B: Control of fetal breathing in the human fetus between 24 and 34 weeks' gestation. Am J Obstet Gynecol 1989;160: 932–938.
41 Walker DW: Effects of increased core temperature on breathing movements and elctrocortical activity in fetal sheep. J Dev Physiol 1988;10:513–523.
42 Suzue T: Respiratory rhythm generation in the in vitro brain stem-spinal cord preparation of the neonatal rat. J Physiol 1984;354:173–183.
43 Smith JC, Greer JJ, Liu G, Feldman JL: Neural mechanisms generating respiratory pattern in mammalian brain stem-spinal cord in vitro. I. Spatiotemporal patterns of motor and medullary neuron activity. J Neurophysiol 1990;64:1149–1169.
44 Dawes GS, Gardner WN, Johnston BM, Walker DW: Effects of hypercapnia on tracheal pressure, diaphragm and intercostal electromyograms in unanaesthetized fetal lambs. J Physiol 1982;326:464–474.
45 Jansen AH, Ioffe S, Russell BJ, Chernick V: Influence of sleep state on the response to hypercapnia in fetal lambs. Respir Physiol 1982;48: 125–142.
46 Kuipers IM, Maertzdorf WJ, Keunen H, De Jong DS, Hanson MA, Blanco CE: Effects of hypercapnia and cold on breathing activity in unanaesthetized fetal lambs in utero. Pediatr Res 1992;31:314A.
47 Ioffe S, Jansen AH, Chernick V: Maturation of spontaneous fetal diaphragmatic activity and fetal response to hypercapnia and hypoxemia. J Appl Physiol 1987;62:609–622.
48 Baier RJ, Hasan SU, Cates DB, Hooper D, Nowaczyk B, Rigatto H: Effects of various concentration of O_2 and umbilical cord occlusion on fetal breathing and behavious. J Appl Physiol 1990;68:1597–1604.
49 Blanco CE, Martin BC, Rankin J, Landauer M, Phernetton T: Changes in fetal organ flow during intrauterine mechanical ventilation with or without oxygen. J Dev Physiol 1988;10:53–62.
50 Tiktinsky MH, Hasan SU, Rigaux A, Bishop B, Morin FC III: The effects of oxygenation on breathing movements in the fetal lamb. Pediatr Res 1992;31:324A.
51 Blanco CE, Chen V, Maertzdorf W, Bamford OS, Hanson M: Effect of hyperoxia (PaO_2 50–90 mm Hg) on fetal breathing movements in the unanaesthetized fetal sheep. J Dev Physiol 1990;14:235–241.
52 Koos BJ, Sameshima H, Power GG: Fetal breathing, sleep state and cardiovascular responses to graded anemia in sheep. J Appl Physiol 1987; 63:1463–1468.
53 Bissonnette JM, Hohimer AR: Acute anemic hypoxemia produces a transient depression in fetal respiratory activity. J Appl Physiol 1987; 63:1942–1946.
54 Koos BJ, Sameshima H, Power GG: Fetal breathing movements, sleep state and cardiovascular responses to an inhibitor of mitochondrial ATPase in sheep. J Dev Physiol 1986;8:67–75.
55 Natale R, Clewlow F, Dawes GS: Measurement of fetal forelimb movements in the lamb in utero. Am J Obstet Gynecol 1981;140: 545–551.
56 Blanco CE, Dawes GS, Walker DW: Effects of hypoxia on polysynaptic reflexes of unanaesthetized fetal and newborn lambs. J Physiol 1983;339: 453–466.
57 Blanco CE, Dawes GS, Hanson MA, McCooke HB: The response to hypoxia of arterial chemoreceptors in fetal sheep and newborn lamb. J Physiol 1984;351:25–37.
58 Moore PJ, Parkes MJ, Noble R, Hanson MA: Reversible blockade of the secondary fall of ventilation during hypoxia in anaesthetized newborn sheep by focal cooling in the brain stem. J Physiol 1991;438: 242P.
59 Koos BJ, Chao A, Doany W: Adenosine stimulates breathing in fetal sheep with brain stem section. J Appl Physiol 1992;72:94–99.
60 Noble R: Brain stem mechanisms mediating the neonatal ventilatory response to hypoxia; in Hanson MA (ed): The fetal and Neonatal Brain Stem: Developmental and Clinical Issues. Cambridge, University Press, 1991, pp 48–58.
61 Johnston BM, Moore PJ, Bennet L, Hanson MA, Gluckman PD: Almitrine mimics hypoxia in fetal sheep with lateral pontine lesions. J Appl Physiol 1990;69:1330–1335.
62 Kuipers IM, Maertzdorf WJ, Keunen H, De Jong DS, Hanson MA, Blanco CE: The effect of maternal hypoxia on unanaesthetized normoxic-hyperoxic fetal lambs. J Physiol 1993;459:334 (abstract).

Biol Neonate 1994;65:189–193

Studies of Neuroregulators in the Brain Stem of SIDS

N. Kopp[a]
L. Denoroy[b]
C. Eymin[a]
N. Gay[a]
F. Richard[a]
K. Awano[a]
R. Gilly[c]
D. Jordan[a]

[a] Laboratoire d'Anatomie Pathologique, Faculté de Médecine A.-Carrel, et
[b] Laboratoire de Médecine Expérimentale, Inserm U52, Unité CNRS URA 1195,
[c] Centre Hospitalier Lyon Sud, Pierre Bénite, Lyon, France

Key Words
Brain stem
Neuroregulators
Sudden infant death

Abstract
Some dysmaturity of neuroregulator neuronal systems may be responsible for brain stem disorders. These disorders may partly explain the mechanism of death in SIDS. The available data using microbiochemical assays, immunocytochemical techniques and autoradiographic methods seem to show anomalies of some monoaminergic and of some peptidergic systems, especially in the medulla oblongata. All these data need to be confirmed by further studies. It should be understood that one positive effect of such neuroanatomical study on SIDS is to gain 'normative' data on the human brain during development.

The brain of SIDS can disclose lesions (inflammatory, ischemic, etc.) at postmortem examination. These lesions can participate in the 'explanation' or 'unexplanation' of sudden infant death.

Underlying brain and/or visceral lesions, there is the possibility of anomalies (maturational?) of different anatomical structures (in the central nervous system, in the peripheral autonomic nervous system, in the viscera with their capters, nerve endings) implicated in the control of vital functions and of sleep-wakefulness states (which are relevant since SIDS strikes in most instances during sleeping periods). Many of these structures are loacted in the brain stem. These possible maturational anomalies are probably subtle if they exist since no clear-cut anatomical lesions have been described like it has been in degenerative diseases as Parkinson's disease.

The maturation of a neuronal system can be addressed by the phenotype appearance (cytoskeleton, etc.), morphology (dendritic spines, etc.) or by the functional cytochemistry of neuroregulators (i.e. neurotransmitters, neuromodulators, neurohormones), their enzymes, their DNA, their binding sites.

The choice of these neuroregulators which are analyzed in a given study is guided by their pharmacological properties on a given function. For instance, substance P is implicated in pain and also has an influence on respiration

N. Kopp
Laboratoire d'Anatomie Pathologique
Faculté de Médecine A.-Carrel
rue Guillaume-Paradin
F–69372 Lyon Cedex 08 (France)

0006–3126/94/
0654–0189$5.00/0

when introduced in certain areas of brain stem with microiontophoresis techniques.

These chemical studies of the brain stem cannot be done on cases that are not well characterized and selected. This would be a loss of energy and time. These chemical studies are to be correlated with morpho-anatomical data: neuronal cell counts, dendritic spines quantification. Astrocytes (which play a major role in the metabolism of some neurotransmitters such as GABA) should also be addressed.

Brain stem is a key area for SIDS studies; hypothalamus probably is too. The brain is not a Russian-doll meccano-like construction. There are no 'centers' in the brain but networks interconnected to each other. All the brain should be ideally studied.

The available data are, after all, fairly rare [1–4].

Catecholaminergic Systems

The activity of DOPA decarboxylase was found to be normal in the SIDS victims medulla and pons [5]. The activity of tyrosine hydroxylase was found to be increased and that of dopamine β-hydroxylase (DBH) to be decreased in the hypothalamus, putamen, and caudate nucleus [5]. Activity in the brain stem was normal suggesting that alteration of catecholamine synthesizing enzymes was not generalized. These studies involved large brain regions rather than discrete nuclei and would have missed focal changes. It is thus possible that anatomically restricted alterations of catecholaminergic systems exist in the brain stem of SIDS victims. We measured the activity of DBH and phenylethanolamine-N-methyltransferase (PNMT) in discrete nuclei of the medulla and pons in victims of SIDS and in controls [6]. PNMT activity was significantly decreased in the Kölliker-Fuse nucleus, the nucleus retroamibugalis and the C2 medullary region (containing the DMV and the NTS). In this latter region, DBH activity was also markedly altered in other areas of the medulla of pons. This work, performed on 10 cases and 6 controls, suggests that alterations in catecholamines synthesizing enzymes may exist and be anatomically restricted in the brain stem of SIDS victims. In a second study of 28 SIDS and 9 controls, PNMT activity was confirmed to be decreased in SIDS victims in the C2 medullary area, the nucleus ambiguus and the nucleus medullae oblongatae centralis [7]. The changes appear to be localized in areas involved in cardiorespiratory control. Since PNMT activity is that most frequently decreased, it may be that central adrenergic neurons are a major site of alterations in SIDS. Furthermore, in 6 cases of SIDS compared to 4 controls, PNMT immunoreactivity was not seen in tyrosine hydroxylase positive neurons of the dorsal part of the NTS [8, 9]. Takashima and Becker [10] showed that the delayed dendritic development of neurons in the ventrolateral medulla implies catecholaminergic neurons. The medulla oblongata adrenaline neurons are known to be involved in autonomic control especially in central regulation of blood pressure [11–13]. A role for central adrenergic neurons in respiratory control has been suggested [14]. The functional significance of the decrease in PNMT activity in SIDS remains to be determined, but the change could underlie alterations in respiratory and cardiovascular controls and in sleep pattern.

Serotonergic Systems

By high-pressure chromatography, we studied the concentration of serotonin (5HT) and its metabolite, 5-hydroxyindole acetic acid (5HIAA) in discrete areas of the raphe microdissected by the punch technique [15]. We compared 4 cases of totally explained sud-

Table 1. 5HT and 5HIAA concentrations (expressed in ng/mg proteins) and 5HT/5HIAA ratio in different raphe areas

	TESID			PESID			USID		
	5HT	5HIAA	5HT/5HIAA	5HT	5HIAA	5HT/5HIAA	5HT	5HIAA	5HT/5HIAA
PA4	n = 3			n = 8			n = 19		
	0.28 ±0.16	1.68 ±1.21	0.23 ±0.15	0.98 ±1.06	1.74 ±1.61	0.58 ±0.55	0.52 ±0.61	1.81 ±0.69	0.33 ±0.39
PA8	n = 4			n = 7			n = 19		
	0.34 ±0.14	1.46 ±0.77	0.26 ±0.11	0.55 ±0.48	1.23 ±0.28	0.46 ±0.44	0.51 ±0.47	1.51 ±0.69	0.34 ±0.24
OB4	n = 4			n = 7			n = 19		
	5.65 ±2.37	5.34 ±2.53	0.94 ±0.4	9.04 ±4.79	7.96 ±2.99	1.2 ±0.7	8.43 ±4.3	8.9 ±2.65	0.97 ±0.41
OB8	n = 4			n = 7			n = 19		
	8.76 ±0.96	17.7 ±5.85	0.54 ±0.19	10.92 ±5.51	15.03 ±6.15	0.68 ±0.25	10.41 ±4.53	17.76 ±7.35	0.63 ±0.3
POV	n = 3			n = 6			n = 19		
	6.24 ±1.46	26.8 ±7.93	0.24 ±0.07	7.99 ±2.33	25.78 ±10.6	0.37 ±0.22	5.91 ±4	25.48 ±9.78	0.21 ±0.09
MA	n = 3			n = 9			n = 19		
	3.51 ±0.73	8.73 ±2.19	0.41 ±0.13	5.01 ±2.28	9.52 ±3.38	0.51 ±0.14	4.98 ±4.56	8.85 ±3.28	0.52 ±0.24

PA = Nucleus raphe pallidus; OB = nucleus raphe obscurus; PO = nucleus raphe pontis; MA = nucleus raphe magnus; V = ventral part. Dissected following Kopp et al. [15]. Mean and SD.

den infant death (TESID), 9 cases of partly explained sudden infant death (PESID) and 19 cases of unexplained sudden infant death (USID) (table 1). Microdissected punches were stored at −20 °C during approximately 12 months (table 1).

No significant difference appeared between the three groups. These data are to be interpreted with extreme caution because of numerous possible sources of artifacts (postmortem delay, anatomical dissection, changes occurring at −20 °C). The 5HT/5HIAA was always inferior to 1. The highest concentration was found in nucleus raphe obscurus in its rostral part (level '8') and in nucleus raphe pontis. If we add to these cases 2 additional cases studied in the same experiment that died non-suddenly (one male neonate of a few hours of life who died of meconial inhalation and one boy who died at 7 months of congenital cardiopathy), an increase appears in the USID group in the rostral part (level '8') of the nucleus raphe obscurus of approximately 80% for 5HT ($p < 0.001$) and 50% for 5HIAA ($p < 0.05$); in the same raphe nucleus, an elevation of 90% of 5HT ($p < 0.02$) appears in the PESID group.

Again, these data are reported mainly because they are the first available on 5HT and 5HIAA in infant brain stem. No conclusion on normality or abnormality can be drawn. If the elevation of 5HT and/or 5HIAA was confirmed, it could suggest an anomaly in the functioning of raphe obscurus neurons. The influence of postmortem delay or age on the concentration of 5HIAA in the rostral part of nucleus raphe obscurus was investigated but failed to reveal any significant correlation. The comparison of the concentration of 5HIAA in nucleus raphe pallidus, caudal level ('4') during the different months of the year seemed to show a peak of maximum in April-May and a minimum between in October and February. Here again this data is purely preliminary.

Peptidergic Systems

Involvement of endogenous opioid systems in SIDS has been suggested by Kuich and Zimmerman [16]. The hypothesis was based on: (a) The known impairment of respiration by excess endorphins [17]. (b) The greater role of endogenous opioids in respiratory control during the perinatal period and infancy [18–20]. (c) Reports suggesting that some apneas in infants could be linked to overfunctioning of the central opioid system [17]. Brandt et al. [21] reported the case of an infant with necrotizing encephalomyelopathy whose apneic spells could be temporarily reversed by naloxone. Furthermore, the endorphin level in cerebrospinal fluid was markedly high and the postmortem delay analysis showed elevated Met- and Leu-enkephalin concentrations in cortical areas. (d) On the higher incidence of SIDS among children of drug-dependent mothers [22].

Increased beta-endorphin levels have been reported in cerebrospinal fluid of near-miss infants [23–25], and in the SIDS postmortem study by Coquerel et al. [26]. In a preliminary study, Pasi et al. [27] measured beta-endorphin and beta-lipoprotein levels in the brain regions of 2 SIDS victims. These were found to be higher in the dorsal part of the pons when compared to adult values. In the absence of normal infants values, it is not possible to determine the significance of this observation. In addition, Bergström et al. [28] found no difference in Met-enkephalin levels in the medulla oblongata and a higher substance P to Met-enkephalin ratio in both medulla oblongata and pons. The significance of this observation is still unclear but could underlie alterations in respiratory control since substance P is likely to be involved in the central control of respiration. With quantitative autoradiography, we assessed somatostatin and neurotensin binding sites in the brain stem of SIDS and found an elevation of neurotensin binding sites especially in the nucleus tractus solitarius with a density similar to two (6 and 7 months of intrauterine life) fetuses. Somatostatin binding sites' density was unchanged [29].

Conclusion

The studies reviewed and reported here need confirmation by further works. They do indicate, taken with other morphological data, that the brain stem is probably not normal in 'SIDS' from the point of view of neuroregulation. The anomalies could be maturational.

The study of brain stem has to be integrated in an approach to other parts of the brain. Energy metabolism should always be addressed. The principal aims of such studies should be normative since so little is known about the structure and chemistry of the human brain during infancy. Only the most reliable tools should be used, especially some molecular biological approaches such as 'in situ hybridization' because SIDS brain is still an evasive 'material' to work on, and because maturational anomalies probably are subtle.

References

1 Denoroy L, Kopp N: Disorders of respiration of central origin and sudden infant death syndrome; in Riederer P, Kopp N, Pearson J (eds): An Intoduction to Neurotransmission in Health and Disease. London, Oxford University Press, 1990.

2 Oehmichen M: Recent neuropathologic research in sudden infant death syndrome: A critical review with special consideration of the brain stem; in Maehly A, Williams RL (eds): Forensic Science Progress 4. Berlin, Springer, 1990, pp 127–137.

3 Kinney HC, Filiano JJ, Harper RM: The neuropathology of the sudden infant death syndrome. A review. J Neuropathol Exp Neurol 1992;51:2: 115–126.

4 Kopp N, Denoroy L, Saint-Pierre G, Jordan D: Les anomalies du système nerveux dans le syndrome de mort subite du nourrisson. Pediatric 1992;47:429–439.

5 Ozand PT, Tyson-Tildon J: Alterations of catecholamine enzymes in several brain regions of victims of sudden infant death syndrome. Life Sci 1983;32:1765–1770.

6 Denoroy L, Kopp N, Gay N, Bertrand E, Pujol JF, Gilly R: Activités des enzymes de synthèse des catécholamines dans des régions du tronc cérébral au cours de la mort subite du nourrisson. CR Acad Sci (Paris) 1980;291:245–248.

7 Denoroy L, Gay N, Gilly R, Tayot J, Pasquier B, Kopp N: Catecholamine synthesizing enzymes activity in brainstem areas from victims of sudden infant death syndrome. Neuropediatrics 1987;18:187–190.

8 Chigr F, Najimi M, Jordan D, Denoroy L, Pearson J, Tommasi M, Gilly R, Kopp N: Absence of adrenergic neurons in medulla oblongata in sudden infant death syndrome. CR Acad Sci (Paris) 1989;309:543–549.

9 Kopp N, Chigr F, Denoroy L, Gilly R, Jordan D: Absence of adrenergic neurons in nucleus tractus solitarius in sudden infant death syndrome. Neuropediatrics 1993;24:25–29.

10 Takashima S, Becker LE: Delayed dendritic development of catecholaminergic neurons in the ventrolateral medulla of children who died of sudden infant death syndrome. Neuropediatrics 1991;22:97–99.

11 Saavedra JM, Grobecker H, Axelrod J: Changes in central catecholaminergic neurons in the spontaneously (genetic) hypertensive rat. Circ Res 1978;42:529–534.

12 Renaud B, Fourniere S, Denoroy L, Vincent M, Pujol JF, Sassad J: Early increase in phenylethanolamine-N-methyltransferase activity in a new strain of spontaneously hypertensive rats. Brain Res 1978;159:149–159.

13 Chalmers JP, Minson J, Denoroy L, Stead B, Howe PRC: Brain stem PNMT neurons and experimental hypertension in the rat. Clin Exp Hypertens 1984;A6:243–258.

14 Champagnat J, Denavit-Saubié M, Henry JL, Leviel V: Catecholaminergic depressant effects on bulbar respiratory mechanisms. Brain Res 1979;160:57–68.

15 Kopp N, Denoroy L, Renaud B, Pujol JF, Tabib A, Tommasi M: Distribution of adrenaline synthesizing enzyme activity in the human brain. J Neurol Sci 1979;41:397–409.

16 Kuich TE, Zimmerman D: Could endorphins be implicated in sudden infant death syndrome? N Engl J Med 1981;304:973.

17 Trippenbach T: Effects of drugs on the respiratory control system in the perinatal period and during postnatal development. Pharmacol Ther 1983;20:307–340.

18 Hazinski TA, Grunstein MM, Schluetter MA, Tooley WH: Effect of Naloxone on ventilation in newborn rabbits. J Appl Physiol Resp Environ Exerc Physiol 1981;50: 713–717.

19 Grunstein MM, Grunstein JS: Maturational effect of enkephalin on respiratory control in newborn rabbits. J Appl Physiol Resp Environ Exerc Physiol 1982;53:1063–1070.

20 Gingras-Leatherman JL, McNamara MC, Lawson EE: Age-dependent influence of hypoxia on methioninenkephalin concentration within rabbit brainstem nuclei. Pediatr Res 1986;20:655–657.

21 Brandt NJ, Terenius L, Jacob BB, Klinken L, Nordius A, Brandt S, Blegvad K, Yssing M: Hyperendorphin syndrome in a child with necrotizing encephalomyelopathy. N Engl J Med 1980;303:914–916.

22 Chavez CJ, Ostrea EM Jr, Stryker JC, Smialek Z: Sudden infant death syndrome among infants of drug-dependent mothers. J Pediatr 1979; 95:407–409.

23 Orlowski JP, Lonsdale D, Denko CW: Beta-endorphin levels in infant apnea syndrome: A preliminary communication. Cleve Clin Q 1982; 49:87–92.

24 Tyson-Tildon J, Roeder LM: In Tyson-Tildon J, Roeder LM, Steinschneider A (eds): Metabolic and Endocrine Aspects of SIDS: An Overview. New York, Academic Press, 1983, pp 243–262.

25 Sankaran K, Hindmarsh KW, Wallace SM, McKay RJ, O'Donnel M: Cerebrospinal fluid and plasma beta-endorphin and concentrations in prolonged infant apnea (near-miss sudden infant death syndrome). Dev Pharmacol Ther 1986; 9:224–230.

26 Coquerel A, Buser M, Tayot J, Pfaff F, Matray F, Proust B: Beta-endorphin and neurotensin in brain stem and cerebrospinal fluid in the sudden infant death syndrome. Neurochem Int 1992;20:97–102.

27 Pasi A, Foletta D, Molz G, Hartmann H, Gramsch C, Mehraein P, Pedrinis E: Regional levels of β-lipoprotein and β-endorphin in the brain and the hypophysis of victims of sudden infant death syndrome. Arch Pathol Lab Med 1983;107: 336–337.

28 Bergström L, Lagercrantz H, Terenius L: Post-mortem analyses of neuropeptides in brains from sudden infant death victims. Brain Res 1984;323:279–285.

29 Chigr F, Jordan D, Najimi M, Denoroy L, Sarrieau A, De Broca A, Rostène W, Epelbaum J, Kopp N: Quantitative autoradiographic study of somatostatin and neurotensin binding sites in medulla oblongata of SIDS. Neurochem Int 1992;20: 113–118.

Biol Neonate 1994;65:194–197

James J. Filiano[a]
Hannah C. Kinney[a, b]

Departments of
[a] Neurology and
[b] Pathology, Children's Hospital
and Harvard Medical School,
Boston, Mass., USA

A Perspective on Neuropathologic Findings in Victims of the Sudden Infant Death Syndrome: The Triple-Risk Model

Key Words
Sudden infant death
Arcuate nucleus
Hypomyelination
Ventilatory dysfunction
Apnea
Prone sleeping
Autonomic dysfunction
Neuropathology
Sleep apnea

Abstract
Neuropathologic studies in SIDS victims support the concept that they are not entirely 'normal' prior to death, but rather possess underlying vulnerabilities which put them at risk for sudden death. This concept forms a key link in a triple-risk model for the pathogenesis of SIDS proposed by us. According to this model, sudden death in SIDS results from the intersection of three overlapping factors: (1) a vulnerable infant; (2) a critical developmental period in homeostatic control, and (3) an exogenous stressor(s). An infant will die of SIDS only if he/she possesses all three factors; the infant's vulnerability lies latent until he/she enters the critical period and is subject to an exogenous stressor. According to this model, heterogeneous disorders may make the infant vulnerable to sudden death during the critical period, as potentially exemplified by two previously reported lesions in SIDS brains (arcuate nucleus hypoplasia and subtle hypomyelination). Nevertheless, the triple-risk model does not preclude the possibility that the majority of SIDS deaths will be explained by a single common pathway upon which multiple stressors impinge to produce sudden death during the critical period.

Introduction

The hypothesis that the sudden infant death syndrome (SIDS) is due to a neural abnormality in cardioventilatory control has generated many neuropathologic studies [1, 2]. The detection of subtle abnormalities in SIDS brains indicates that not all SIDS victims are 'normal' despite their lack of clinical abnormalities. The occurrence of brain abnormalities supports the concept that a vulnerable and not a normal infant is at risk for SIDS.

James J. Filiano, MD
Department of Pediatrics (Intensive Care/Neurology)
Children's Hospital at Dartmouth
1 Medical Center Drive
Lebanon, NH 03756 (USA)

0006–3126/94/
0654–0194$5.00/0

The idea of a vulnerable infant forms a key part of a triple-risk model proposed here for the pathogenesis of SIDS. This model is supported by epidemiologic, physiologic, and general autopsy data, as well as concepts presented in the SIDS literature over the last 20 years [1–8]. It differs from other models by its emphasis on neuropathologic findings and the bias that these findings are not incidental.

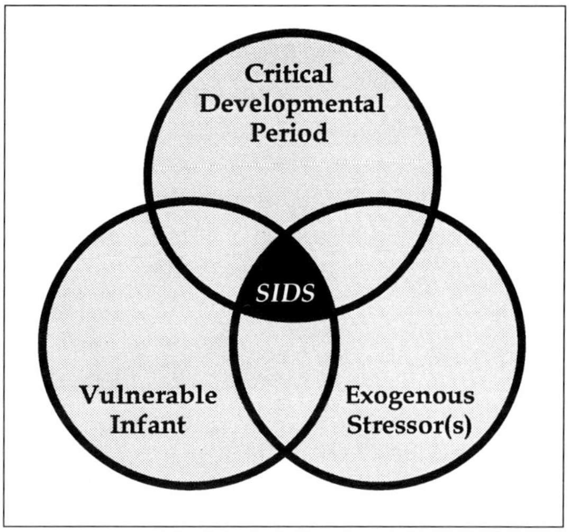

Fig. 1. The Venn diagram of three overlapping circles depicts the triple-risk model of SIDS. According to this model, SIDS results from the intersection of three overlapping factors: (1) underlying vulnerability in the infant; (2) a critical developmental period in homeostatic control; and (3) an exogenous stressor(s).

The Triple-Risk Model of SIDS

The triple-risk model proposes that sudden death in SIDS results from the intersection of three overlapping factors: (1) a vulnerable infant; (2) a critical developmental period for homeostatic control, and (3) an exogenous stressor(s) (fig. 1). According to this model, an infant will die of SIDS only if he/she possesses all three factors; the infant's vulnerability lies latent until he/she enters a critical developmental period and is subject to an exogenous stressor which matches the infant's underlying vulnerability and overwhelms an already compromised homeostatic system. Potentially, heterogeneous disorders may make the infant vulnerable to sudden death during the critical period.

The concept of the vulnerable infant is supported by four lines of evidence: (1) subtle CNS and/or systemic abnormalities in SIDS victims, detected by quantitative or rigorous methods at autopsy; (2) neonatal abnormalities in neurological or autonomic function in at least some infants who subsequently die of SIDS; (3) postneonatal abnormalities in cry, cardiac and ventilatory patterns, and state organization in some future SIDS victims, and (4) maternal and pregnancy-related factors associated with increased SIDS risk [1]. Epidemiologic risk factors include prematurity, low birth weight, young maternal age, maternal anemia, maternal urinary tract infection, and maternal cigarette smoking, opioid use, or cocaine use during pregnancy. Together, these risk factors point to a suboptimal intrauterine environment, and suggest that the mechanisms for risk for SIDS develop in fetal life in at least some cases [1].

The concept of a critical developmental period is based on the consistent age distribution for SIDS [1]. Ninety percent of deaths occur in the first 6 months, with a peak at 2–4 months and a relative sparing of the first month. The triple-risk model addresses this common link by emphasizing the importance of physiologic changes which occur normally during this age range. During this period, major changes occur in virtually all physiologic systems as infants attain adaptive mechanisms enabling them to maintain homeostasis. These changes include dramatic transitions in homeostatic systems regulated by the brain, notably autonomic control, ventilation, sleep-waking state organization, temperature regulation, and circadian rhythms [1]. Although changes in cardiopulmonary function and state organization continue throughout life, a relatively stable configuration is achieved by the end of the first 6 months of life [1, 9]. During this same period, the brain undergoes spectacular developmental changes, with an almost doubling of overall weight [1]. Given the complexity, rapidity, and extent in brain growth, and inherent instability in the rapid transitions in homeostatic control, subtle perturbations may be devastating [1]. The concept that an external stressor precipitates sudden death is derived from epidemiologic studies indicating that minor respiratory or gastrointestinal illness occurs around the time of death in the majority of SIDS victims [10]. Other potential stressors linked to SIDS include fever, hyperthermia induced by over-blanketing, and prone sleeping position [10–12].

The triple-risk model proposes that infants who eventually die of SIDS may appear normal clinically, but their vulnerability lies latent until they enter the critical developmental period between 1 and 6 postnatal months and are subject to an exogenous stressor which overwhelms already compromised cardioventilatory or other homeostatic controls. According to this model, SIDS victims are not 'normal', yet, death occurs only if all three factors intersect and only if the exogenous stressor matches the specific vulnerability of the individual infant (e.g. fasting or a catabolic state in medium chain acyl-Coa dehydrogenase deficiency). By corollary, the infant may survive as 'normal' if the stressor is avoided, or if the underlying vulnerability is ameliorated by therapeutic interventions. Any disruption of transitions in autonomic, ventilatory, temperature, or state regulation may render an infant's homeostatic control even more unstable. In this way, the triple-risk model helps explain the apparently asymptomatic behavior of most SIDS victims prior to death, and helps explain why eliminating an external stressor, e.g. prone sleeping position, may reduce the incidence of SIDS [12]. Given that the stressor must match the infant's vulnerability, the model helps explain why the same stressor is not present in every case, exemplified by recognition that SIDS victims die in both prone and supine positions, and the overwhelming majority of infants who sleep prone do not die of SIDS.

Neuropathologic Findings and the Triple-Risk Model

Neuropathologic research has focused on neural systems that mediate cardioventilatory control. Recent interest has also addressed systems which regulate arousal and its associated cardiopulmonary defense mechanisms [1]. From the perspective of the triple-risk model, in one subset of SIDS victims a brain abnormality may be directly responsible for cardioventilatory and/or arousal dysfunction. In a different SIDS subset, the brain abnormality may be caused by the same basic defect that is responsible for sudden death, although the brain abnormality itself may not be responsible for death, i.e. the brain abnormality is an epiphenomenon of the primary defect. If SIDS victims are made vulnerable by heterogeneous disorders, it is not unexpected that brain abnormalities are not present in all SIDS victims, nor are the same abnormalities necessarily present in every case. Arcuate nucleus hypoplasia in a subset of SIDS victims is a potential example whereby a SIDS victim's brain abnormality may be the underlying vulnerability directly related to death by disrupting cardioventilation and arousal [13, 14]. A subtle delay in myelination in a different subset of SIDS victims [15], on the other hand, may not be directly responsible for sudden death, but rather, a secondary consequence of a lipid or amino acid disorder that results in both sudden death through systemic energy failure and in hypomyelination through defective myelin synthesis.

Conclusion

The potential value of the triple-risk model is that it reconciles seemingly contradictory data in the SIDS literature: SIDS has characteristics of a collection of heterogeneous disorders because a population of SIDS victims contains infants with a variety of underlying vulnerabilities; SIDS has characteristics of a disorder with a single underlying mechanism because of the key influence the critical period has on homeostasis; and, lastly, SIDS has characteristics of a random process affecting normal infants because ostensibly 'normal' infants harbor underlying vulnerabilities, but those who die of SIDS are the ones who undergo the random, fatal intersection of vulnerability, critical period, and stressor. Nevertheless, the triple-risk model does not preclude the possibility that the majority of SIDS deaths will be explained by a single common pathway upon which multiple stressors impinge to produce sudden death during a critical developmental period. If this proves true, the triple-risk model may serve as a frame of reference to help explain the timing of death. Ultimately, it may be necessary to understand all three factors – the vulnerable infant, critical period, and exogenous stressors – in order to prevent SIDS.

References

1 Kinney HC, Filiano JJ, Harper RM: The neuropathology of the sudden infant death syndrome: A review. J Neuropathol Exp Neurol 1992;51: 115–126.
2 Becker LE: Neural maturational delay as a link in the chain of events leading to SIDS. Can J Neurol Sci 1990;17:361–371.
3 Bergman AB: The 'Discovery' of Sudden Infant Death Syndrome: Lessons in the Practice of Political Medicine. Seattle, University of Washington Press, 1986, pp 1–189.
4 Willinger M: SIDS: A Challenge. J NIH Res 1989;1:73–80.
5 Lipsitt LP: Developmental jeopardy in the first year of life: Behavioral considerations; in: Issues in Child Health and Adolescent Health. Hillsdale, Lawrence Erlbaum, 1982, pp 23–37.
6 Hunt CE, Brouillette RT: Sudden infant death syndrome: 1987 perspectives. J Pediatr 1987;110:669–678.
7 Schwartz PJ, Southall DP, Valdes-Dapena M (eds): The sudden infant death syndrome: Cardiac and respiratory mechanisms and interventions. Ann NY Acad Sci 1988;533: 1–474.
8 Harper RM: State-related physiological changes and risk for the sudden infant death syndrome. Aust Paediatr J 1986;(suppl):55–58.
9 Chugani HT, Phelps ME, Mazziotta JC: Positron emission tomography study of human brain functional development. Ann Neurol 1987;22: 48–97.
10 Hoffman HJ, Damus K, Hillman L, Krongrad E: Risk factors for SIDS. Results of the National Institute of Child Health and Human Development SIDS cooperative epidemiology study; in Schwartz PJ, Southall DP, Valdes-Dapena M (eds): The Sudden Infant Death Syndrome. Cardiac and Respiratory Mechanisms and Interventions. Ann NY Acad Sci 1988;533:13–30.
11 Kemp JS, Thach B: Sudden death in infants sleeping on polystrene-filled cushions. N Engl J Med 1991;324: 1858–1864.
12 Guntheroth WG, Spiers PS: Sleeping prone and the risk of sudden infant death syndrome. JAMA 1992;287:2359–2382.
13 Filiano JJ, Choi JC, Kinney HC: Candidate cell populations for respiratory chemosensitive fields in the human infant medulla. J Comp Neurol 1990;293:448–465.
14 Filiano JJ, Kinney HC: Arcuate nucleus hypoplasia in the sudden infant death syndrome. J Neuropathol Exp Neurol 1992;51:394–403.
15 Kinney HC, Brody BA, Finkelstein DM, Vawter GF, Mandell F, Gilles FH: Delayed central nervous system myelination in the sudden infant death syndrome. J Neuropathol Exp Neurol 1991;50:29–48.

Biol Neonate 1994;65:198–204

M. Bonora
M. Boule
H. Gautier

Laboratoire de Physiologie Respiratoire, Faculté de Médecine St-Antoine, Paris, France

Ventilatory Strategy in Hypoxic or Hypercapnic Newborns

Key Words
Control of ventilation
Maturation
Diaphragmatic activity
Metabolism
Sleep state

Abstract
In conscious newborns, the ventilatory response to hypoxia is characterized by precocious hyperventilation followed by tardive hypoventilation, the latter disappearing with age. The hypoventilation could be mainly related to a weak peripheral drive and to the persistence of the diaphragmatic activity during expiration. Also, a decrease in metabolic rate and body temperature interferes with the response. The hyperventilation in response to hypercapnia increases as maturation proceeds and the maturation of the peripheral chemoreceptors contribute to this effect, as during hypoxia. The responses to both stimuli depend on many factors such as sleep state, anesthesia or ambient temperature.

The regulation of breathing during the neonatal period undergoes dramatic changes with the maturation of the neurophysiological, metabolic and mechanical components of the respiratory control system. The respiratory activity in response to hypoxia, hyperoxia or hypercapnia varies therefore with gestational and postnatal ages, but also with size and maturity at birth of each species. In addition, sleep state which affects several respiratory reflexes and muscle activities certainly plays an important modulating role in the control of breathing of the newborn.

Ventilatory Response to Hypoxia

In contrast to the adult, the newborn is generally unable to sustain an increase in ventilation in response to hypoxia. The inhalation of a hypoxic gas mixture induced in most newborns a transient hyperventilation during the first minute followed by a sustained reduction in ventilation towards or even below normoxic baseline levels. This biphasic response has been shown in preterm and term humans and in different animal species such as monkeys, piglets, lambs, kittens and rabbits, in conscious as well as in anesthetized newborns [1, 2]. However, larger and precocial species re-

Dr. M. Bonora
Faculté de Médecine St-Antoine
Laboratoire de Physiologie Respiratoire
27, rue de Chaligny
F–75012 Paris (France)

0006–3126/94/
0654–0198$5.00/0

spond to hypoxia by a sustained increase in ventilation even in their early life [3].

The initial increase in ventilation is brought about by an increase in tidal volume (VT) and frequency (f), while the subsequent decrease in ventilation is due to a large decrease in VT in spite of an increase in f in conscious animals [1, 4] and mainly to a large decrease in f in anesthetized animals [5].

With increasing gestational age, the initial hyperventilation is more pronounced in newborn infants, but the late hypoventilation does not seem to change [6]. With increasing postnatal age, the initial hyperventilation has been found to increase also in newborn monkeys, lambs and kittens [1, 2], but not in newborn infants [6], while the late hypoventilation is progressively replaced by a sustained hyperventilation. Such an adult-like response is observed at various ages depending on the degree of maturity of the species, between a few days after birth in precocial animals as in lambs [7] to a few weeks in altricial animals as in kittens [4].

The mechanisms underlying these ventilatory changes are not yet fully understood. It has been suggested that the fall in ventilation in young newborns may be related to several factors such as a reduction in dynamic lung compliance, or to the hypoxia-induced changes in concentration of several endogenous mediators related to the respiratory activity such as endorphins, adenosine, GABA, serotonin and catecholamines. But, most studies have focused on the maturation of peripheral and central chemoreceptors. Indeed, although peripheral chemoreceptors have been found to be active in the fetus and at birth [8], their relatively weak activity may not be sufficient enough to counterbalance the hypoxic depression originating from the central nervous system. This hypothesis has been supported by the fact that such rapid shallow breathing elicited by moderate levels of hypoxia in unanesthetized kittens [4] is also observed during central hypoxia induced in newborn lambs breathing low levels of carbon monoxide [9] or in adult cats either after carotid-body denervation or also during CO hypoxia [10]. The forebrain structures have been suggested to be involved in this tachypneic breathing since it cannot be elicited in decerebrated adult cats [10] or rabbit pups [11] and, moreover, it shares several common features with thermal panting which depends upon the hypothalamic thermoregulatory centers.

To test the hypothesis that the hypoxic hypoventilation was centrally mediated, some authors have recorded the diaphragmatic electromyographic activity in unanesthetized hypoxic newborns as an index of central respiratory activity. It was shown that the large reduction in tidal volume in response to hypoxia was paradoxically associated with an elevated diaphragmatic activity implying that the mechanisms involved in late decreased ventilation with hypoxia were rather located in the lung or in the respiratory pump.

However, the difference observed between the central output and ventilation during hypoxia may also be explained by an increase in end-expiratory lung volume which can be mainly induced by increasing either the post-inspiratory activity of the diaphragm or the laryngeal resistance. Such a braking mechanism at the diaphragmatic level has already been observed in human infants during normoxia [12].

We have therefore suggested that this phenomenon could also occur in newborns during hypoxia and, in a recent study, we have examined the response to steady state hypoxia on the whole diaphragmatic activity and ventilation in conscious 2-week-old kittens [13]. We have shown that when kittens are breathing 10% O_2, the peak activity of the diaphragm at the end of inspiration was effectively increased while tidal volume was greatly reduced, but the diaphragmatic activity persisted throughout expiration and therefore remained higher than baseline at the end of expiration. Thus, the differential activity of the diaphragm between the end of expiration and the next inspiration which represents the phasic activation of the diaphragm was decreased by hypoxia and was well matched with the reduced tidal volume.

These findings suggested therefore that in addition to the weakness of the peripheral drive, a central mechanism should also participate in the resopnse to hypoxia in newborns.

Such a phenomenon has also been found in older animals [13]. This postinspiratory activity of the diaphragm is therefore an important mechanism used by young and older conscious newborns to reduce the action of the central inspiratory drive during hypoxia by braking the expiratory airflow. This control of expiratory airflow has also been observed during hypercapnia in adult cats in which, on the contrary, the braking mechanisms are inhibited to speed expiration so that a larger VT is exhaled in a shorter period of time [14]. During hypoxia, the persistent activity of the diaphragm up to the end of expiration should increase the functional residual capacity (FRC). Indeed, such raised FRC above resting volume has been reported in newborn lambs and monkeys [15] and the postinspiratory activity of inspiratory muscles contributes to this effect, even though a laryngeal braking due to narrowing of the vocal cords likely plays a major role in this phenomenon [15]. Such increased FRC which should increase the oxygen stores is possibly beneficial to the newborn.

Ventilatory Response to Hyperoxia

The administration of high levels of oxygen induces the reverse effects of hypoxia, with a transient decrease in ventilation followed by a return to baseline or by a slight hyperventilation as found in newborn infants [6]. The initial hypoventilation increases with postnatal age [7, 16], while the secondary hyperventilation has been found to be similar in young and older newborn infants [6]. The steady state response to hyperoxia has been rarely studied, but the small increase in ventilation observed in young infants could be explained by the central stimulating effect of oxygen previously shown in carotid body denervated adult cats [17].

Ventilatory Response to Hypercapnia

Newborn mammals, including infants, respond to CO_2 by a sustained hyperventilation [2, 18]. A brisk increase in ventilation mediated by the peripheral chemoreceptors appears within 3–5 s and a secondary increase in ventilation begins 25–30 s later [19]. The initial hyperventilation results from an increase in both VT and f, while the late response is achieved through a marked increase in VT with minimal changes in f.

The CO_2 sensitivity which is characterized by the slope and the intercept of the CO_2 response curve has been reported to increase with advancing gestational age in infants [20], but not in primates [21].

During postnatal life, the CO_2 sensitivity increases during the first month in preterm infants and in both premature and full-term primates [20, 21], although in puppies, the percent changes in ventilation in response to a low level of CO_2 (2%) does not change between 2 weeks and 4 months of age [22]. Similarly, we have found in a recent work that in 16 conscious kittens, the ventilatory response to 3 and 5% CO_2 increases between 2 and 4 weeks of age (fig. 1). Indeed, the percent increase in ventilation when breathing 5% CO_2 as compared to air breathing was 128 ± 63%

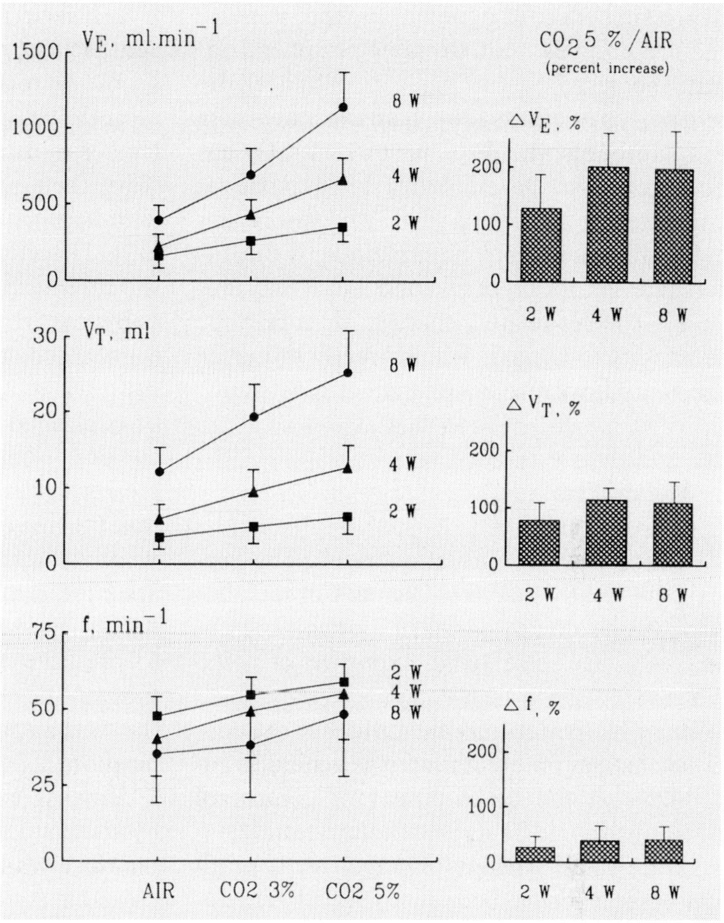

Fig. 1. Left: Mean values (± SD) of minute ventilation ($\dot{V}_E$), tidal volume (V_T) and respiratory frequency (f) in response to 3 and 5% inspired CO_2 in 2-, 4-, and 8-week-old kittens. Right: Percent increase in the ventilatory components in response to 5% CO_2 as compared to air breathing at different ages.

($\bar{x}$ ± SD) at 2 weeks and 202 ± 77% at 4 weeks, while at 8 weeks of age, the percent increase remains stable (199 ± 84%).

The contribution of peripheral drive in this response in relation with maturation has recently been shown by Marchal et al. [23] who found that the carotid chemoreceptor response to hypercapnia was present but small in magnitude in young newborn kittens and developed with age. To determine the central component of the ventilatory response to hypercapnia, experiments can be performed under hyperoxia which greatly reduced the chemoreceptor activity. However, the interpretation of results is difficult since, as mentioned above, hyperoxia by itself has a depressing effect on the peripheral chemoreceptor activity and a stimulating effect on central respiratory activity [17].

The interaction between the response to hypercapnia and hypoxia in newborns and its postnatal evolution is not yet clearly analyzed. In young infants or monkeys, the ventilatory response to steady state hypercapnia decreases with hypoxia as compared to air [24, 25]. This type of negative interaction between hypercapnia and hypoxia has been explained as being the result of a predominant central depressing effect of hypoxia. Indeed, in more mature animals with stronger peripheral input, the response to CO_2 was enhanced by hypoxia as in adults [26]. However, in young immature rats, the response to 10% CO_2 has been found to be enhanced by hypoxia as compared to hyperoxia [18]. The discrepancies in the results may be explained by the different levels of CO_2 or O_2 used, but it may also reflect species-related changes in metabolic sensitivity to hypoxia which greatly influence the ventilatory responses to chemical stimuli.

Metabolism

The changes in ventilation induced by hypoxia are tightly linked to changes in metabolism, which already varies in room air breathing with age, size, cold exposure or sleep state.

In order to minimize the influence of metabolic changes on breathing, it is generally admitted that the development of control of breathing should be studied at the neutral temperature range whereby metabolism is minimal while a normal body temperature is maintained. But, it should be pointed out that (1) normal body temperature of newborns in their early life is generally lower than that kept by adults; (2) the thermoneutral range which is poorly defined should be carefully adjusted to the age for each species, and (3) neutral temperature for metabolism is not necessarily the neutral or optimal temperature regarding the respiratory function for newborns, especially when they have to face a slight heat stress as their heat loss mechanisms are poorly efficient. In fact, the ambient temperature in the nest of most newborns is likely to be below the thermoneutral range and the use of high environmental temperatures leads to artificial conditions and may induce severe respiratory disturbances such as tachypnea [27] or apnea [28].

It has been suggested that the decrease in ventilation during hypoxia in newborns should be related to the decrease in metabolic rate, the drop in $\dot{V}O_2$ during hypoxia being greater in a relatively cool environment [29]. Nevertheless, the lowering of O_2 consumption with hypoxia occurs also at thermoneutrality [30]. Therefore, a decrease in metabolic rate should interfere with the ventilatory response to hypoxia. In fact, the decrease in ventilation is not associated to a rise in $PaCO_2$ but, on the contrary, to a decrease [30]. These results can be explained by the fact that the drop in O_2 consumption induced by hypoxia is much greater than the drop in ventilation, implying that the newborn may rather relatively hyperventilate during hypoxia. Hence, it can be assumed that the decrease in metabolic rate during hypoxia may be a part of the strategy to preserve arterial PO_2, and it emphasizes the importance of the metabolic adaptation in the ventilation response to hypoxia of the newborn.

Finally, exposure to hypoxia induced, in newborns, a substantial decrease in body temperature which progressively waned with increasing age [27, 30]. It has been shown recently that this hypoxia-induced fall in body temperature (BT) results from, and does not contribute to the decrease in metabolic rate [31]. Such decreased body temperature in hypoxia has been considered as a new set point of thermoregulation lower than in normoxia, since an external warming to restore the normoxic BT level results in a relatively hyperthermic situation with an increase in ventilation without changing the hypometabolism. Thus, there is a tight coupling between changes in metabolism and ventilation during hypoxia in the newborn which seems to choose to protect the arterial PO_2 by decreasing energy utilization and temperature homeostasis.

Sleep State

The profound influence of behavioral states on eucapnic ventilation and respiratory control have been thoroughly examined only in the last decade and further studies are necessary to clarify this important subject.

The incidence of REM sleep on different mechanisms involved in the regulation of breathing is especially determinant during the postnatal period since newborns spend most of their time in this sleep state. Indeed, the typical paradoxical breathing observed in newborns due to their high chest wall compliance is enhanced during REM sleep mainly because of a marked inhibition of tonic and phasic intercostal muscle activities [32]. Also, the expiratory braking mechanisms which increase the functional residual capacity are altered during REM sleep since the laryngeal adductor activity and postinspiratory activity of the diaphragm are inhibited [16].

The influence of sleep on the ventilatory response to hypoxia and hypercapnia is not quite clearly established and the results seem to depend mostly on the technique used. In fact, when the progressive rebreathing technique is used, the response to both stimuli is generally decreased in REM sleep as compared to NREM sleep. But with the steady state method, the response to hypercapnia is similar in both sleep states, but the response to hypoxia is increased during REM sleep and decreased during NREM sleep.

Also, the arousal reflex from sleep which is considered an important defense mechanism initiated by different respiratory stimuli is not similar in both sleep states. During both hypoxia and hypercapnia, arousal is delayed during REM sleep compared to NREM sleep, and during hypoxia, it occurs at much lower SaO_2 in REM sleep. This reflex which could be mainly mediated by the peripheral chemoreceptors [33] may represent a crucial problem in young newborns with weak peripheral drive, especially during REM sleep.

It seems, therefore, that in addition to the specific ventilatory sensitivity to hypoxia, hyperoxia or hypercapnia, the variability in the respiratory activity observed in newborns depends upon several factors, such as the degree of maturity at birth of the species, the gestational and postnatal ages, but also the effect of anesthesia, sleep state, ambient temperature, methods used, level and duration of the stimulus. Finally, secondary effects may influence the ventilatory response, such as the changes in metabolism, body temperature and state of consciousness induced by the stimulus. For the interpretation of the results, all these factors should be, if not kept under control, at least kept in mind.

References

1 McCooke HB, Hanson MA: Respiration of conscious kittens in acute hypoxia and effect of almitrine bismesylate. J Appl Physiol 1985;59:18–23.

2 Steele AM: Developmental changes in neural control of respiration; in Gootman YM (ed): Developmental Neurobiology of the Autonomic Nervous System. Clifton, Humana Press, 1986, pp 327–401.

3 Mortola JP, Rezzonico R, Lanthier C: Ventilation and oxygen consumption during acute hypoxia in newborn mammals: A comparative analysis. Respir Physiol 1989;78:31–43.

4 Bonora M, Marlot D, Gautier H, Duron B: Effects of hypoxia on ventilation during postnatal development in conscious kittens. J Appl Physiol 1984;56:1464–1471.

5 Blanco CE, Hanson MA, Johnson P, Rigatto H: Breathing pattern of kittens during hypoxia. J Appl Physiol 1984;56:12–17

6 Rigatto H, Brady JP, Chir B, de la Torre Verduzco R: Chemoreceptor reflexes in preterm infants: I. The effect of gestational and postnatal age on the ventilatory response to inhalation of 100% and 15% oxygen. Pediatrics 1975;55:604–613.

7 Bureau MA, Begin R: Postnatal maturation of the respiratory response to O_2 in awake newborn lambs. J Appl Physiol 1982;52:428–433.
8 Blanco CE, Dawes GS, Hanson MA, McCooke HB: The response to hypoxia of arterial chemoreceptors in fetal sheep and newborn lambs. J Physiol (Lond) 1984;351:25–37.
9 Bureau MA, Carroll JL, Canet E: Response of newborn lambs to CO-induced hypoxia. J Appl Physiol 1988;64:1870–1877.
10 Gautier H, Bonora M: Possible alteration in brain monoamine metabolism during hypoxia-induced tachypnea in cats. J Appl Physiol 1980;49:769–777.
11 Martin-Body RL, Johnston MA: Central origin of the hypoxic depression of breathing in the newborn. Respir Physiol 1988;71:25–32.
12 England SJ, Kent G, Stogryn HAF: Laryngeal muscle and diaphragmatic activities in conscious dog pups. Respir Physiol 1985;60:95–108.
13 Bonora M, Boule M, Gautier H: Diaphragmatic and ventilatory response to alveolar hypoxia and hypercapnia in conscious kittens. J Appl Physiol 1992;72:203–210.
14 Gautier H, Remmers JE, Bartlett D Jr: Control of the duration of expiration. Respir Physiol 1973;18:205–221.
15 Cote AK, Yunis PW, Mortola JP, Bureau MA: Dynamics of breathing in the hypoxic awake lambs. J Appl Physiol 1988;64:354–359.
16 Hertzberg T, Hellstrom S, Lagercrantz H, Pequignot JM: Development of the arterial chemoreflex and turnover of carotid body catecholamines in the newborn rat. J Physiol (Lond) 1990;425:211–225.
17 Gautier H, Bonora M: Effects of hypoxia and respiratory stimulants in conscious intact and carotid denervated cats. Bull Eur Physiopathol Resp 1982;8:565–582.
18 Saetta M, Mortola JP: Interaction of hypoxic and hypercapnic stimuli on breathing pattern in the newborn rat. J Appl Physiol 1987;62:506–512.
19 Carroll JL, Canet E, Bureau MA: Dynamic ventilatory responses to CO_2 in the awake lamb: Role of the carotid chemoreceptors. J Appl Physiol 1991;71:2198–2205.
20 Rigatto H, Brady JP, de la Torre Verduzco R: Chemoreceptor reflexes in preterm infants. II. The effect of gestational and postnatal age on the ventilatory respone to inhaled carbon dioxide. Pediatrics 1975;55:614–621.
21 Guthrie RD, Standaert TA, Hodson WA, Woodrum DE: Development of CO_2 sensitivity: Effects of gestational age, postnatal age, and sleep state. J Appl Physiol 1981:50:956–961.
22 Haddad GG, Leistner HL, Epstein RA, Epstein MAF, Grodin WK, Mellis RB: CO_2-induced changes in ventilation and ventilatory pattern in normal sleeping infants. J Appl Physiol 1980;48:684–688.
23 Marchal F, Bairam A, Haouzi P, Crance JP, Di Giulio C, Vert P, Lahiri S: Carotid chemoreceptor response to natural stimuli in the newborn kitten. Respir Physiol 1992;87: 183–185.
24 Rigatto H, Kalapesi Z, Leathy FN, Mccallum M, Cates D: Ventilatory response to 100% O_2 and 15% O_2 during wakefulness and sleep in preterm infants. Early Hum Dev 1982; 7:1–10.
25 Guthrie RD, Laframboise WA, Standaert TA, Van Belle G, Woodrum DE: Ventilatory interaction between oxygen and carbon dioxide in the preterm primate. Pediatr Res 1985;19:528–533.
26 Purves MJ: The respiratory response of the newborn lamb to inhaled CO_2 with and without accompanying hypoxia. J Physiol (Lond) 1966;185:78–94.
27 Bonora M, Gautier H: Maturational changes in body temperature and ventilation during hypoxia in kittens. Respir Physiol 1987;68:359–370.
28 Hey EN, Katz G: The optimum thermal environment for naked babies. Arch Dis Childh 1970;45:328–334.
29 Hill JR: The oxygen consumption of new-born and adult mammals. Its dependence on the oxygen tension in the inspired air and on the environmental temperature. J Physiol (Lond) 1959;149:346–373.
30 Mortola JP, Rezzonico R: Metabolic and ventilatory rates in newborn kittens during acute hypoxia. Respir Physiol 1988;73:55–68.
31 Pedraz C, Mortola JP: CO_2 production, body temperature, and ventilation in hypoxic newborn cats and dogs before and after body warming. Pediatr Res 1991;30:165–169.
32 Henderson-Smart DJ, Read DJC: Depression of intercostal and abdominal muscle activity and vulnerability to asphyxia during active sleep in the newborn; in Guilleminot C, Dement WC (eds): Sleep Apnea Syndromes. New York, Liss, 1978, pp 93–117.
33 Fewell JE, Kondo CS, Dascalu C, Filyk SC: Influence of carotid denervation on the arousal and cardiopulmonary response to rapidly developing hypoxemia in lambs. Pediatr Res 1989;25:473–477.

Biol Neonate 1994;65:205–210

Teresa Trippenbach

Department of Physiology, McGill University, Montreal, Canada

Pulmonary Reflexes and Control of Breathing during Development

Key Words

Slowly adapting mechanoreceptors
Rapidly adapting mechanoreceptors
C fibres
Vagal stimulation
Lactic acid

Abstract

The potency of the Hering-Breuer inspiratory-inhibitory and expiratory-promoting reflexes decreases with maturation in mammals. The Hering-Breuer deflation reflex is present at birth and its power changes little during postnatal development. Already during the second day of life the airway defence reflex resembles that of the adult rabbits. In contrast, sensitivity of the pulmonary chemoreflex does not reach the adult level by the end of the first week of life in newborns of the same species. The time course of functional development of respiratory reflexes coincides with the maturity of different species at birth.

Development of vagal respiratory reflexes matches rapid changes that take place in the central and peripheral nervous systems after birth. Four main sets of vagal reflexes have been described in adult mammals: (1) the Hering-Breuer inflation reflexes (expiratory-promoting and inspiratory-inhibitory); (2) the Hering-Breuer deflation reflex; (3) the airway defence reflex, and (4) the pulmonary chemoreflex.

The Hering-Breuer Inflation Reflexes

Two types of vagal slowly adapting mechanoreceptors are present in adult animals: low threshold receptors which are active at end expiratory volume, and high threshold receptors which are activated only at volumes above functional residual capacity (FRC). In contrast in newborns, slowly adapting activity is present only during inspiration [1, 2]. However, despite the sparse activity, the Hering-Breuer inflation reflexes are more powerful in the newborn than they are in adult mammals [3, 4]. Therefore, in contrast to the adult human [5], in newborn infants during eupnea, the Hering-Breuer inspiratory-inhibitory reflex may affect the depth and duration of inspiration.

The Hering-Breuer expiratory promoting reflex becomes stronger towards the end of expiration in adult [6, 7] and newborn [8] animals. In the adults, inputs coming at delays exceeding 80% of the control expiratory time, fail to have an effect. It is believed that the last

Dr. T. Trippenbach
Department of Physiology, McGill University
McIntyre Medical Sciences Bldg
3655 Drummond Street
Montreal, PQ H3G 1Y6 (Canada)

0006–3126/94/
0654–0205$5.00/0

20% of expiratory phase represents activation time of the inspiratory on-switch mechanism [9]. In the majority of newborns, the end-expiratory insensitive phase is missing, and the stronger response to both vagal [8] and intercostal muscle stimulation [10] occurs at the longest stimulus delays. Variations in the time course of the expiratory response in newborns imply that if the end-expiratory insensitive phase is present during the early postnatal life, it could be affected by body temperature, chemical drive, and anesthesia. This is in contradiction to the adult cats which show a stable insensitive fraction of expiration under different experimental conditions [6, 7]. If under certain conditions the irrevocable period of expiration is indeed absent in newborns, the respiratory phase-switching mechanism may be open to influences from peripheral and central inputs throughout the total respiratory cycle. This may represent one of the possible sources of instability of the pattern of breathing in newborns.

The Hering-Breuer Deflation Reflex

Data in the literature imply that in various mammalian species during the first 2 weeks of life, slowly adapting mechanoreceptors are the only vagal receptors present during the early postnatal life [1, 2]. Accordingly, a decrease in FRC would decrease already sparse vagal phasic volume-related activity, and a decrease in FRC and vagotomy should have qualitatively similar respiratory effects in newborns. To challenge this hypothesis we tested the respiratory effects of changes in FRC and vagotomy in rabbits during the first 4 days of life [11]. Elevation of FRC had no effect on inspiration and the diaphragmatic EMG, and triggered the Hering-Breuer expiratory-promoting reflex. These effects suggest that already at birth, tonic vagal slowly adapting mechanoreceptors are able to exert selective control over expiratory duration. Lowering FRC evoked an increase in inspiratory activity and a shortening of both timing phases, but mainly expiration. These results suggest activation of the Hering-Breuer deflation reflex [12, 13]. Similar effects of lung deflation were recorded in newborn kittens and monkeys [4]. In contrast to lung deflation, vagotomy induced a prolongation of both timing phases, and an increase in peak amplitude of inspiratory activity without affecting its rate of rise [11]. The discrepancy between effects of lung deflation and vagotomy suggests that lung deflation triggered a vagally mediated excitation. The origin of this excitation is obscure.

Two groups of vagal receptors have been proposed to be involved in the deflation reflex in adult animals, i.e. rapidly adapting mechanoreceptors [12], and specific, deflation-sensitive receptors [13]. In newborns, the deflation receptors have not yet been defined, and activity of rapidly adapting mechanoreceptors has been reported to be absent until the second week of life in puppies [2]. In adult dogs tachypnea may be recorded in response to right ventricular distention which can be elucidated by application of the negative pressure to the airways [14]. Hence, vagal cardiac receptors should also be considered as one of the pathways which can affect the respiratory pattern already during the early postnatal life. Low activity and yet a strong reflex suggests high sensitivity of the respiratory controller to either of these inputs already at birth.

The Airway Defence Reflex

Our results suggest that sensitivity of the airway defence reflex rapidly increases during the first week of life in rabbits [15]. In awake 1-day-old pups neither breathing dust nor his-

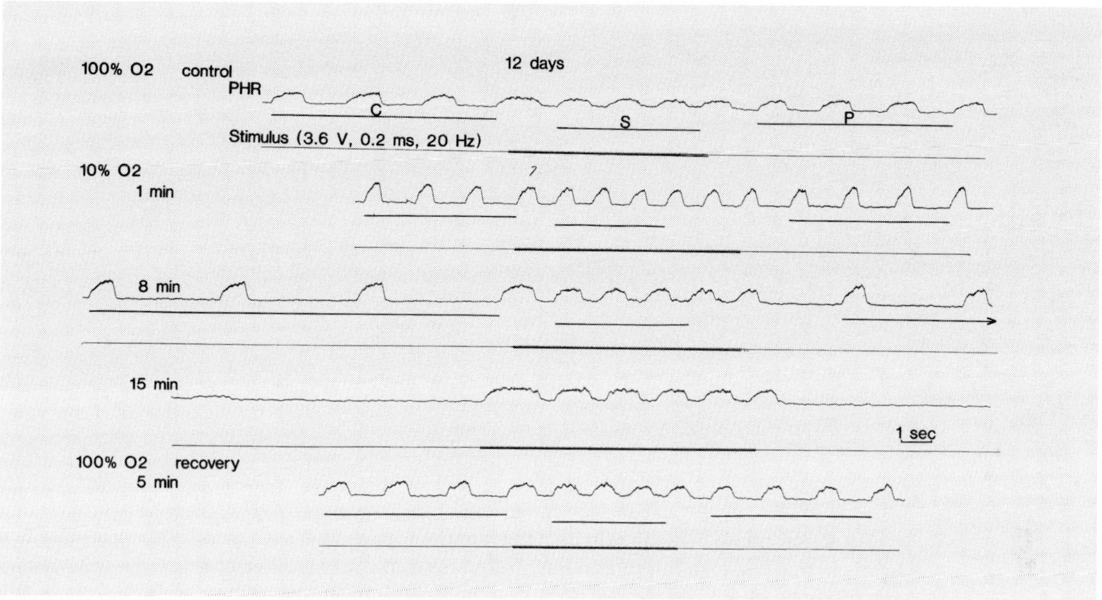

Fig. 1. Example of response of integrated phrenic activity (PHR) to vagal stimulation recorded in a urethane-anesthetized, paralyzed and artificially ventilated 12-day-old rabbit. Stimulation, with parameters indicated in the figure, was applied during control (ventilation with 100% O_2), hypoxia-evoked respiratory excitation (ventilation with 11% O_2 balanced N_2), hypoxia-evoked respiratory depression and apnea, and during recovery after hypoxia (ventilation with 100% O_2). Time from the onset of hypoxic run and recovery at which stimulation was applied is indicated to the right of the figure. Horizontal lines mark control (C), stimulated (S), and poststimulation (P) phrenic cycles.

tamine aerosol had effects. However, already during the second day of life both stimuli provoked rapid and shallow respiration that is typical for the airway defence reflex in the adult animals. Injection of histamine into the pulmonary circulation confirmed low sensitivity of this reflex immediately after birth in rabbits. In 2-day-old and older rabbits histamine increased peak amplitude of the diaphragmatic EMG, peak tracheal pressure and respiratory rate, and decreased tidal volume. The increase in both, the pressure and inspiratory activity, and a decrease in tidal volume suggests that histamine produced airway constriction and decreased dynamic lung compliance. These effects of histamine are typical for the adult animals [16]. In contrast, in 1-day-old rabbits histamine provoked an increase in both the EMG and tidal volume. The age-dependent effects of histamine may rely on a low number of rapidly adapting mechanoreceptors and sparsity of bronchial smooth muscle fibres after birth [17]. Presence of the histamine-evoked rapid and shallow breathing in 2-day-old newborns suggests the intense developmental changes in the rabbit's lung tissue that take place during the first 2 days of life.

Vagally mediated respiratory excitation might be important for preservation of the respiratory rhythm in newborns. Figure 1 shows an example of the effects of vagal stim-

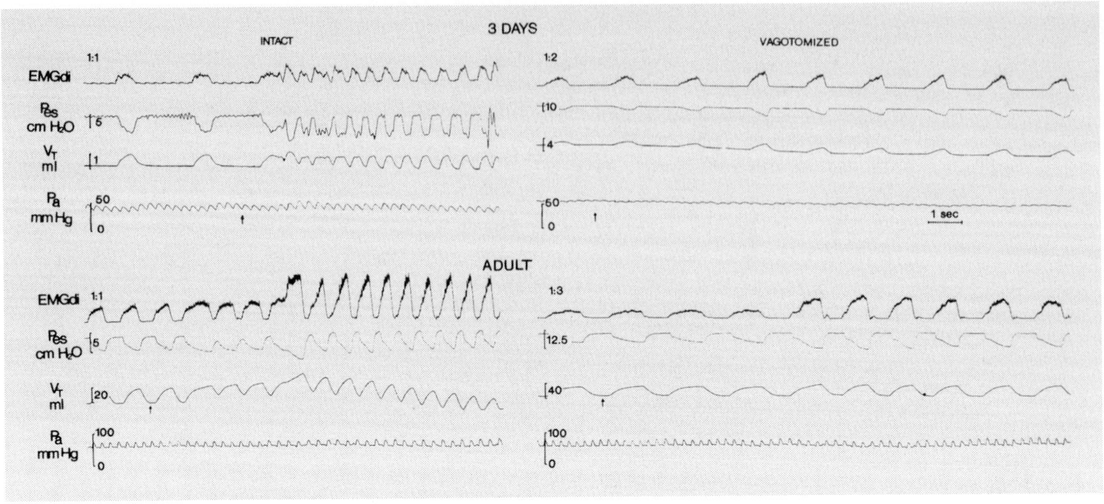

Fig. 2. Response to lactic acid injected into the jugular vein before and after vagotomy in a 3-day old pup and an adult rabbit. Early response (rapid and shallow breathing) is followed by late response characterized by deep and fast respiration. Vagotomy abolished the early response in both animals. In the adult rabbit, a dose of 0.25 m*M*/kg was given. In the newborn the dose of lactic acid had to be doubled to evoke the early response. Time scale is the same in all records. Arrows indicate time of injection. In the EMG trace ratios 1:1, 1:2, and 1:3 show different attenuation factors. Modified from Ducros and Trippenbach [23].

ulation, with pulses of low frequency and high amplitude, during control, hypoxia-evoked respiratory excitation and depression, and finally hypoxic apnea in an anesthetized, vagotomized and artificially ventilated 12-day-old rabbit. Despite hypoxia-evoked respiratory inhibition, the respiratory rate acceleration produced by vagal stimulation was similar at each of these conditions in this and all other pups from the 1st to 14th day of age.

The Pulmonary Chemoreflex

The pulmonary chemoreflex is mediated by nonmyelinated vagal fibres, C fibres [18, 19]. The reflex cannot be activated by phenyl diguanide in kittens younger than 6 days of age [20]. In contrast, a fully developed cardiorespiratory response to right atrial injection of the same chemical was present in 2-day-old piglets [21].

Pulmonary edema, pulmonary vascular prominence, and local hyperinflation of the lung are pathological changes which produce tachypnea via stimulation of pulmonary C fibres in adult animals [19]. These pathological changes are present in infants with the transient tachypnea syndrome after birth. Gradual decrease in breathing frequency to normal levels has a time course similar to that of clearing the roentgenographic abnormalities [22]. Therefore, it is possible that already at birth C fibres may affect the breathing pattern in infants. To test this hypothesis, we examined the respiratory effect of stimulation of C fibres by lactic acid [18] injected into the pulmonary circulation in newborn and adult rabbits [23]. Figure 2 illustrates example of effects of lactic acid on the diaphragmatic EMG, tidal volume, esophageal and blood pressures, before and after vagotomy in a 3-day-old and an adult rabbit. In both animals, lactic acid induced an increase in the rate of breathing and in FRC. However, the threshold dose of lactic acid for the adult animals had to be doubled to produce a similar effect in the 3-day-old and older rabbits during the first week of life. A further increase in the dose was necessary to produce parallel effects in 1- and 2-day-old newborns. The early excitatory effects were always followed by a long-lasting increase in frequency, tidal volume and the diaphragmatic EMG. After vagotomy the early respiratory excitation was abolished, and the following, long-lasting effects remained unchanged. High threshold of the early response suggests immaturity of at least one of the components of the reflex feedback loop involved in the respiratory effects of lactic acid during the 1st week of life in rabbits. This is in agreement with a study on kittens [20] but they are in contrast to a study on newborn piglets [21]. The difference in the excitability of this reflex response may coincide with the greater maturity of pigs than cats and rabbits at birth. Therefore, C fibres should be taken into account as one possible factor contributing to transient tachypnea syndrome in infants.

In summary, despite increasing activity of slowly adapting mechanoreceptors, the Hering-Breuer inspiratory inhibitory and expiratory promoting reflexes lose their strength during postnatal development. The end-expiratory insensitive phase is absent during the first 2 weeks of postnatal life in rabbits. The lack of the end-expiratory insensitive phases may represent one of the possible sources of instability of the respiratory pattern in newborns. Despite the reported absence of vagal rapidly adapting mechanoreceptors, the Hering-Breuer deflation reflex is present already at birth in various mammalian species. Sensitivity of the airways defence reflex progressively increases during the first week of life in rabbits. Sensitivity of the pulmonary chemoreflex does not reach its adult level by the end of the first week of life in rabbits. However, because of different maturity of different species at birth, the C fibres may be involved in the tachypnea syndrome in infants.

Acknowledgments

Research presented here was supported by the Hospital for Sick Children Foundation, Toronto, Canada, and the MRC of Canada.

References

1 Schwieler GH: Respiratory regulation during postnatal development in cats and rabbits and some of its morphological substrate. Acta Physiol Scand 1968;304(suppl):3–123.

2 Fisher JT, Sant'Ambrogio G: Location and discharge properties of respiratory vagal afferents in newborn dog. Respir Physiol 1982;50:209–220.

3 Bodegard G, Schwieler GH, Skoglund S, Zetterstrom R: Control of respiration in newborn babies. I. The development of the Hering-Breuer inflation reflex. Acta Physiol Scand 1969;58:567–571.

4 Trippenbach T, Zinman R, Mozes R, Murphy LM: Differences and similarities in the control of breathing pattern in the adult and neonate; in von Euler C, Lagercrantz H (eds): Central Nervous Control Mechanisms in Breathing. Oxford, Pergamon Press, 1979, pp 313–326.

5 Clark FJ, von Euler C: On the regulation of depth and rate of breathing. J Physiol 1972;222:267–295.

6 Knox CK: Characteristics of inflation and deflation reflexes during expiration in the cat. J Neurophysiol 1973;36:284–295.
7 von Euler C, Trippenbach T: Temperature effects on the inflation reflex during expiratory time in the cat. Acta Physiol Scand 1976;96:338–350.
8 Trippenbach T, Kelly G: Expiratory effects of vagal stimulation in newborn kittens. J Appl Physiol 1985;59:218–222.
9 Feldman JL, Gautier H: Interaction of pulmonary afferents and pneumotaxic center in control of respiratory pattern in cats. J Neurophysiol 1976;39:31–44.
10 Trippenbach T, Kelly G, Marlot D: Respiratory effects of stimulation of intercostal muscles and saphenous nerve in kittens. J Appl Physiol 1983;54:1736–1744.
11 Trippenbach T, Kelly G, Marlot D: Effects of tonic vagal input on breathing pattern in newborn rabbits. J Appl Physiol 1985;59:223–228.
12 Sellick H, Widdicombe JG: Vagal deflation and inflation reflexes mediated by lung irritant receptors. Q J Exp Physiol 1970;55:153–163.
13 Koller EA, Ruegg DG, Ferrer P: Approach to a quantitative differentiation between the respiratory effects evoked from the lung stretch and the lung deflation receptors during thoracic compression. Experientia 1971;27:163–164.
14 Kostreva DR, Hopp FA, Zuperku EJ, Kampine JP: Apnoea, tachypnea, and hypotension elicited by cardiac vagal afferents. J Appl Physiol 1979;47:312–318.
15 Trippenbach T, Kelly G: Respiratory effects of cigarette smoke, dust, and histamine in newborn rabbits. J Appl Physiol 1988;64:837–845.
16 Sellick H, Widdicombe JG: Stimulation of lung irritant receptors by cigarette smoke, carbon dust, and histamine aerosol. J Appl Physiol 1971;31:15–19.
17 Thurlbeck WM: Postnatal growth and development of the lung. Am Rev Respir Dis 1975;111:803–844.
18 Trenchard D: Chemoreflex in rabbits. Respir Physiol 1986;66:367–386.
19 Coleridge HM, Coleridge JCG, Schultz HD: Afferent pathways involved in reflex regulation of airway smooth muscles. Pharmacol Ther 1989;41:1–63.
20 Kalia M: Visceral and somatic reflexes produced by J pulmonary receptors in newborn kittens. J Appl Physiol 1976;41:1–6.
21 Schleman M, Gootman N, Gootman PM: Cardiovascular and respiratory responses to right atrial injections of phenyl diguanide in pentobarbital-anesthetized newborn piglets. Pediatr Res 1979;13:1271–1274.
22 Kuhn JP, Fletcher BD, de Lemos RA: Roentgen findings in transient tachypnea of the newborn. Radiology 1969;92:751–757.
23 Ducros G, Trippenbach T: Respiratory effects of lactic acid injected into the jugular vein of newborn rabbits. Pediatr Res 1991;29:548–552.

Biol Neonate 1994;65:211–219

Christian F. Poets[a]
Martin P. Samuels[b]
David P. Southall[b]

[a] Department of Paediatric Pulmonology, Medizinische Hochschule, Hannover, FRG;
[b] Academic Department of Paediatrics, North Staffordshire Hospital Centre, University of Keele, Stoke-on-Trent, UK

Epidemiology and Pathophysiology of Apnoea of Prematurity

Abstract

In preterm infants, reliance on the detection of apnoeic pauses and/or bradycardia results in significant amounts of hypoxaemia remaining undetected. In addition, recordings of breathing movements and ECG do not have predictive value for subsequent sudden infant death. In recent years, the ability to continuously monitor and record arterial oxygen saturation (SaO_2) has produced important information regarding the mechanisms for respiratory events in the preterm population. Normal data on SaO_2 (Nellcor N-200) and breathing movements have been collected in 160 preterm infants. Median baseline SaO_2 during regular breathing was 99.5% (range 88.7–100) at the time of discharge from SCBU and 100% (95.3–100) at follow-up 6 weeks later. Episodic desaturations ($SaO_2 \leq 80\%$ for ≥ 4 s) ranged between 0 and 355 episodes per 12-hour recording. In a study of a separate group of 16 preterm infants with recurrent cyanotic episodes of unknown cause, the total number of abnormal hypoxaemic episodes was markedly increased. These hypoxaemic episodes were associated with three breathing pattern: (i) absent breathing movements; (ii) continued breathing movements, but absent airflow, and (iii) continuous airflow and breathing movements. Thus, preterm infants with cyanotic episodes have an increased number of clinically unapparent hypoxaemic episodes, some of which occur with continued breathing and airflow. In another study of 79 patients who had been born preterm and had a history of an apparent life-threatening event, 43 (54%) had abnormal oxygenation on multichannel recordings, including 23% with clinically undetected baseline hypoxaemia. Continuous additional inspired oxygen was given to 27 patients with recorded abnormalities in oxygenation and a history of recurrent ALTE needing cardiopulmonary resuscitation: in 25, episodes stopped or markedly reduced in frequency. Home PO_2 monitoring has been undertaken in 73 patients for a median duration of 7.1 months. Recognition and treatment of abnormalities in episodic or baseline hypoxaemia may reduce the risk for recurrent cyanotic episodes or subsequent apparent life-threatening events at home. In infants with a history of such episodes, the use of additional inspired oxygen and home PO_2 monitoring are helpful in management. The finding of abnormal hypoxaemia may be relevant to the increased risk of sudden death found in preterm infants.

Key Words

Apnoea of prematurity
Preterm infants
Hypoxemia
Pulse oximetry

Prof. D.P. Southall
Academic Department of Paediatrics
North Staffordshire Hospital Centre
Hartshill, Stoke-on-Trent ST4 (UK)

0006–3126/94/
0654–0211$5.00/0

Definition

The definition of apnoea of prematurity has changed considerably over the years. In particular, the minimum duration used to define clinically significant apnoea decreased from 2 min in 1956 [1] to 20 s in 1978 [2]; in some studies, it has since become even shorter [3]. The Task Force on Prolonged Apnea of the American Academy of Pediatrics has defined pathological apnoea when there is 'cessation of breathing for 20 s or longer, or as a brief episode if associated with bradycardia, cyanosis, or pallor' [2]. This definition was the first to acknowledge the difficulties involved in separating physiologic from pathologic apnoea: it is not the apnoea per se, but its potential effects on circulation and/or on blood gas homeostasis, particularly oxygenation, that might be harmful to the infant, and it is not only a cessation of breathing efforts that may cause severe hypoxaemia or cyanosis, but a whole variety of different mechanisms, including upper and lower airway obstruction and ventilation/perfusion mismatch. In this review, we will therefore concentrate predominantly on the incidence and pathophysiology of disturbances in oxygenation rather than on apnoeic pauses, regarding the latter as only one amongst several mechanisms that may cause hypoxaemia in preterm infants.

Incidence of Apnoea

Daily et al. [4] observed apnoeic pauses of 20 s or longer in 13 of 22 infants (59%) with birthweights of between 765 and 2,552 (mean 1,417) g, who were monitored during their first 1–2 weeks of life. Alden et al. [5] reported an incidence of 84% for apnoeic pauses of 30 s or longer in a study on 161 infants of birthweights less than 1,000 g. Henderson-Smart [6] observed an inverse relationship between the proportion of infants having 3 or more apnoeic pauses of >20 s in duration and gestational age: 7% of infants born at 34–35 weeks' gestation had recurrent apnoea, compared with 54% of those born at 30–31 weeks' gestation, and up to 78% of those born at 26–27 weeks' gestation. In the latter study, apnoeas commenced in 77% of infants within their first 2 days of life; they had ceased by 37 weeks post-conceptional age in 92%, and by 40 weeks in 98% of infants.

Incidence of Episodes of Hypoxaemia

As mentioned above, it is not the apnoeic pause, but its effect on oxygenation that is relevant to the well-being of the preterm infant. Until the introduction of transcutaneous oxygen monitoring, the recognition of sudden episodic hypoxaemia relied exclusively on the observation of cyanosis, which inevitably is highly subjective. The degree of hypoxaemia at which cyanosis occurs is also variable, depending on factors such as haemoglobin levels and skin blood flow. With the introduction of transcutaneous oxygen ($TcPO_2$) monitors, clinicians became aware that preterm infants may exhibit episodes of hypoxaemia (defined as $TcPO_2 < 40$ mm Hg) which can occur without a cessation of breathing movements and even without a cessation of airflow [7, 8]. However, $TcPO_2$ values depend not only on arterial oxygenation, but also on cardiac output and skin perfusion, and a severe fall in $TcPO_2$ may thus occur without a corresponding change in arterial PO_2. Therefore, objective information about the frequency of intermittent dips in *arterial* oxygenation has only become available with the introduction of pulse oximetry. The latter method allows a reliable, continuous and non-invasive measurement of arterial oxygenation which is almost independent of cardiac output or skin perfusion, provided that the

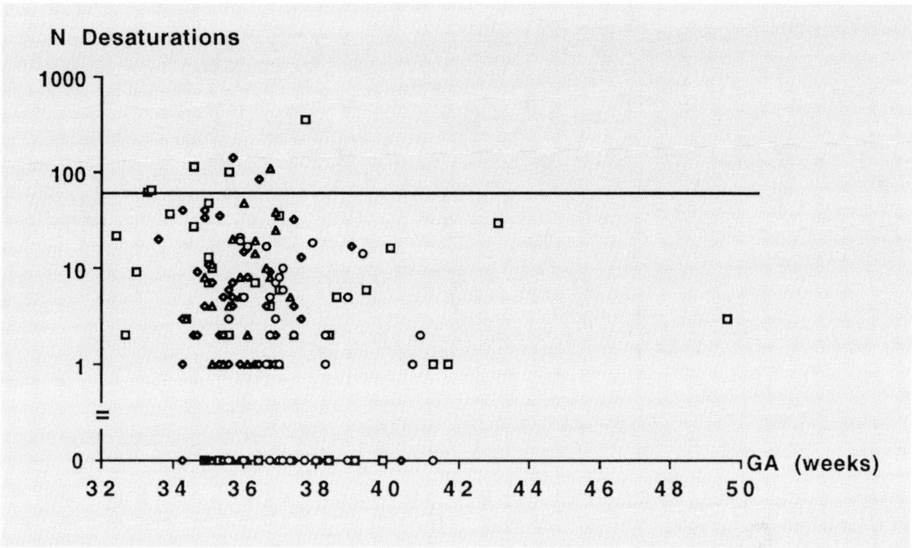

Fig. 1. Number of episodes of desaturation per recording from 160 preterm infants at the time of discharge from hospital, corrected to a mean duration of recording of 12.2 h and plotted against GA at recording ($r = -0.2$, $p < 0.05$). Note the logarithmical scale on the y axis. Symbols as in figure 2. The horizontal line represents the 95th centile for all recordings (61 episodes per 12.2 h of recording). From Poets et al. [10], with permission.

make of oximeter has been previously validated against arterial line measurements in infants and young children [9].

We have recently obtained data on baseline oxygen saturation (SaO_2) and on the frequency and duration of episodes of desaturation in 160 preterm infants at the time of their discharge from hospital, using the Nellcor N100 with N200 software in the beat-to-beat mode [10]. The infants had a mean gestational age of 32.8 (SD 2.5) weeks at birth, and of 36.6 (SD 2.1) weeks when studied. In the full-term infant, episodic falls in SaO_2 to 80% or less (desaturations) are common, but usually short; 97% are shorter than 4 s [11]. In the preterm infants [10] we concentrated only on relatively prolonged episodes of desaturation, i.e. on those in which SaO_2 remained at or below 80% for at least 4 s. We found such episodes of desaturation in 114 (71%) of the 160 12-hour overnight recordings, with a median frequency of 3 episodes per recording, and a median duration of 5.3 s. Only 8% of episodes (in 48 recordings) lasted for longer than 10 s. A minority of infants showed extremely frequent desaturation, which had not been recognised clinically (all had been considered ready for discharge); one infant had 355 episodes of desaturation in her recording (the 95th centile was 61, fig. 1). Interestingly, 6 of the 8 infants with values above the 95th centile had not reached term (GA ≥ 37 weeks) at the time of study.

Although episodic desaturation was apparently more common in the preterm infants than in those born at term, most (91%) of the former had baseline saturations, measured during quiet sleep, which were in the same range as previously described for full-term infants, i.e. above 97% [10, 11]. The median

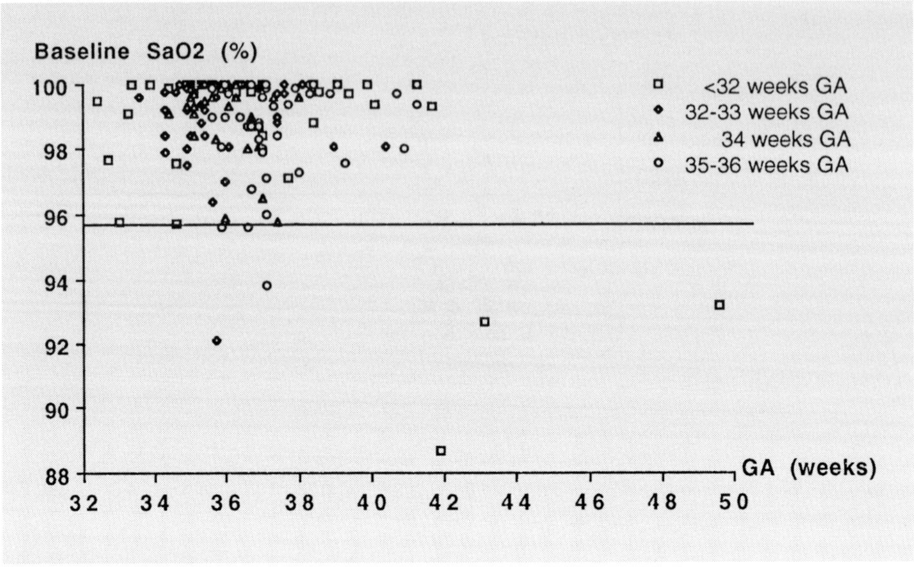

Fig. 2. Baseline SaO_2 in recordings as in figure 1 (n = 160), plotted against GA at recording (r = –0.1, p = 0.3). The horizontal line represents the 5th centile for baseline SaO_2 in all 160 recordings (95.7%). From Poets et al. [10], with permission.

baseline SaO_2 was 99.5%. A minority, however, had a clinically unrecognised low baseline SaO_2 (lowest 88.7%, 5th centile 95.7%, fig. 2). Again, none of these infants had been clinically considered hypoxaemic, and all were breathing room air at the time of study.

One hundred and ten infants from the above study [10] underwent a follow-up recording at around 6 weeks following their discharge recording. At follow-up, all of the outlying results observed at discharge had normalised: the lowest baseline SaO_2 was now only 95.3% (5th centile 97.9%), and the highest number of episodic desaturations was 17 (95th centile 3 episodes of desaturation per recording). A comparison with a group of full-term infants of comparable gestational age (42–47 weeks) showed that the preterm infants had a significantly higher baseline SaO_2, and no more desaturation, than the infants born at term.

These data show that self-resolving falls in SaO_2 to 80% or less, lasting for 4 s or longer, are a common phenomenon in preterm infants even at a time when they are clinically considered well and ready for discharge from the hospital. These data may also provide a guideline to separate 'normal' from 'abnormal' episodic and baseline hypoxaemia in this age group. However, they do not provide information about outcome, and do thus not provide a basis for the decision as to whether an abnormal degree of hypoxaemia in an infant otherwise considered well should be treated or not. Nevertheless, there is good evidence that hypoxaemia has potentially deleterious effects on development and may be a cause of sudden death [12–14], and it has therefore become our policy to temporarily increase the concentration of inspired oxygen in those infants who demonstrate abnormal hypoxaemia in an overnight recording, particularly as our follow-up data show that such treatment will usuallly only be required for a few weeks.

Pathophysiology of Apnoea and Hypoxaemia in Preterm Infants

Although our understanding of the pathophysiology of apnoeic/cyanotic episodes in preterm infants is growing, there are yet several questions which remain unanswered. These include (1) whether or not differences in the breathing patterns observed during these episodes imply that there are differences in their underlying pathophysiology; (2) whether the airway closure observed during some episodes occurs at the level of the pharynx, the larynx, the lower airways, or at some combination of the three; (3) whether this airway closure is an active or a passive process; (4) whether non-apnoeic mechanisms may contribute to the hypoxaemia observed during these episodes, and (5) whether the frequent occurrence of apnoeic/cyanotic episodes in preterm infants reflects an immaturity of their central nervous system, their lung mechanics, or both. This review will concentrate on these questions.

Three different types of apnoeic pauses have been identified from recordings of breathing movements and nasal/oral airflow. These include prolonged apnoeic pauses (called 'central' apnoea), which are characterised by a cessation of both respiratory efforts and airflow, episodes of absent airflow, but continued breathing movements (called 'obstructive' apnoea), and a combination of the two above (called 'mixed' apnoea). The relative frequency of these 3 patterns varies between studies, depending on the minimum durations used to define an apnoeic pause and on the age of the infants studied. For example, Waggener et al. [15], including all apnoeic pauses of ≥ 3 s duration, found that 55% were 'central', 31% 'mixed', and 14% 'obstructive'. In contrast, Upton et al. [16], including only pauses that lasted for at least 5 s, observed 58% 'central', 35.5% 'mixed', and 6.5% 'obstructive' apnoeic pauses, whereas the corresponding figures given in a study by Butcher-Puech et al. [17], who used an even longer minimum pause duration (10 s), were 69, 20 and 11%, respectively.

The descriptive finding of differences in airflow and breathing movement patterns during different apnoeic episodes may imply that these reflect different disease entities. However, more detailed studies suggested that the clear distinction between 'central', 'obstructive' and 'mixed' apnoeas cannot be maintained. Thus, Milner et al. [18] suggested back in 1980 that airway closure may not only occur during 'obstructive', but also during 'central' apnoeic pauses. More recently, Upton et al. [16] observed signs of airway closure in the majority of apnoeic episodes in preterm infants, including those which were apparently solely 'central'. Waggener et al. [15] analysed oscillations in breath-by-breath ventilation of preterm infants, and observed that 'central', 'mixed' and 'obstructive' apnoeic pauses all occurred at the minimum phase of spontaneous ventilatory oscillations, suggesting that all 3 patterns had one common component. Whether an apnoeic pause was 'central' or 'obstructive' would, according to these authors, only 'be determined by the relative drive to the diaphragm as compared with the muscles of the oropharynx' [15].

The latter speculation implies that the maintenance of airway patency, not its interruption, is an active process. This hypothesis is based on (1) the observation that oropharyngeal obstruction may occur during general anaesthesia in adults, and (2) autopsy studies in young infants, which showed that in natural resting postures the upper airways were closed, suggesting that a neuromuscular mechanism is necessary to maintain airway patency during life [19]. This hypothesis, however, has been challenged in a recent study from Ruggins and Milner [20], who used fibreoptic nasendoscopy to examine the pharynx and larynx during apnoeic episodes in preterm infants, and described an *active* laryngeal closure in association with apnoea. They suggested that this was possibly caused by the laryngeal chemoreflex.

Similar controversy exists with regard to the site of airway obstruction. Mathew et al. [21] used a saline-filled catheter, connected to a pressure transducer, to determine the level of airway obstruction in 9 preterm infants with clinical apnoea. They found that the level of obstruction was almost always in the upper pharynx. In contrast, Ruggins and Milner [20] in their above study involving fibreoptic nasendoscopy only observed *hypo*-pharyngeal, i.e. laryngeal closure. We have observed, however, major hypoxaemic episodes in both preterm infants and older infants with severe cyanotic breath-holding continue despite bypass of both the pharynx and the larynx by tracheal intubation [22]. This suggests either that there was not only upper, but also lower airway obstruction [22], or that the pharyngeal or laryngeal closure was a secondary response to disturbances in the periphery of the lung. The latter mechanism has been proposed by Stransky et al. [23], who observed apnoea, bradycardia and laryngeal closure after pharmacological stimulation of pulmonary C fibres. Physiologically, these fibres are stimulated by an increase in pulmonary interstitial pressure, as occurs is in pulmonary edema, or during a deep inspiration (e.g. a sigh) [24].

Sudden severe hypoxaemia may also develop without a cessation in either breathing movements or airflow (fig. 3). Such episodes have been observed in preterm infants with recurrent cyanotic episodes of unknown cause [25], in term infants with respiratory tract infections [26], and also in asymptomatic preterm infants [27]. In the first group, measurements of the slope of desaturation during episodes with continued ventilation showed that hypoxaemia progressed 2–3 times faster than during isolated apnoeic pauses in the same infant [25]. This latter observation makes it extremely unlikely that the desaturations despite continuous breathing were solely due to hypoventilation; they are more likely to result from a sudden intrapulmonary shunt [22].

Non-apnoeic mechanisms contributing to apnoea-induced hypoxaemia have also been demonstrated during periodic apnoea in preterm infants. We measured the slope of desaturation during hypoxaemic episodes associated with this breathing pattern, and found it faster for periodic than for non-periodic apnoeic pauses in the same infant (median 8.4%/s during periodic vs. 4.3%/s during non-periodic apnoea, $p < 0.005$) [28]. The more rapid desaturation in periodic apnoea could not be explained by a decrease in baseline SaO_2 between desaturations, or an increase in oxygen consumption. These differences in the slope of desaturation between the two breathing patterns could indicate changes in ventilation/perfusion matching, perhaps triggered by airway hypoxia or by intermittent falls in lung volume below closing volume during the repeated apnoeic pauses [22, 29].

Does the frequent occurrence of apnoeic/cyanotic episodes in preterm infants reflect an immaturity of the central nervous (brain stem) centres involved in the regulating of breathing, or an immaturity in lung mechanics? The former hypothesis is apparently supported by observations of prolonged apnoeic pauses and the presence of longer brain stem conduction times from auditory evoked responses in preterm infants with 'apnoea' compared with controls [30]. Preterm infants, in contrast to older infants, also respond to hyp-

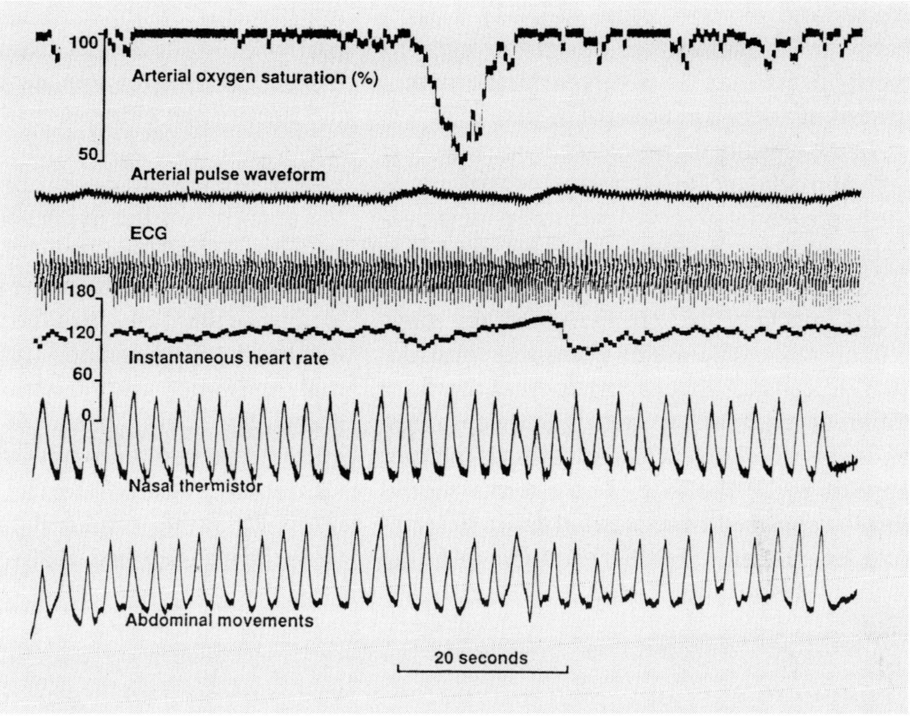

Fig. 3. Section from a multichannel physiologic recording, showing an episode of desaturation with continued breathing. There is a fall in SaO_2 to 50%, lasting 12 s, which occurs without any significant change in either breathing movements or nasal airflow. From Poets et al. [22], with permission.

oxia with a sustained *de*crease, not increase, in ventilation, a response which again suggests an immaturity of central chemoreceptors [31]. Nevertheless, there are also data to suggest that apnoeic/cyanotic episodes are not just caused by a switching-off of the central generator(s) of inspiratory activity. For example, Fleming et al. [32] observed apnoea lasting up to 20 s after stimulation of irritant receptors in the carina of preterm infants; older infants (> 35 weeks GA) responded to the same stimulus with an *increase* in inspiratory effort. Heldt [33] demonstrated a relationship between chest wall instability and apnoea in preterm infants. Thibeault et al. [29] observed some 25 years ago that recurrent apnoeic pauses may be abolished by increasing functional residual capacity via the application of negative extrathoracic pressure. The same effect can also be achieved by continuous positive airway pressure (CPAP) [34]. The striking effects of CPAP on the frequency of apnoeic/hypoxaemic episodes in preterm infants has led to suggestions that 'the apnoea in these infants may be related to a decreasing lung volume and increasing intrapulmonary shunt' [34], i.e. it may be triggered by intermittent airway closure (atelectasis) resulting from the highly compliant chest wall with resultant afferent activity producing apnoeic pauses and airway closure [23, 32]. Hence, peripheral (lung) as well as central nervous mechanisms may be involved in the pathogenesis of apnoea in preterm infants.

In conclusion, we believe that both apnoeic and non-apnoeic mechanisms contribute to the hypoxaemia observed during apnoeic/cyanotic episodes in preterm infants, and that peripheral (lung) as well as central (brain stem) mechanisms are involved in their pathogenesis. The use of terms like 'obstructive' or 'central' apnoea implies that there are different mechanisms causing these episodes, and that these are clearly defined; neither appears to be the case. These terms should thus be replaced by somewhat more descriptive expressions. Further studies into the mechanisms leading to these episodes, and in particular to the airway closure so frequently associated with the apnoea, are required. In the light of the evidence summarised in this review, the term 'apnoea of prematurity' may also be somewhat inappropriate, as it is not the apnoea, but the hypoxaemia that is most relevant to both the well-being of the infant and the understanding of the pathophysiology leading to these episodes. To establish criteria for the identification and treatment of abnormal episodic and baseline hypoxaemia, knowledge about normal oxygenation is required. Such data are now available for preterm infants at around term, and we are currently obtaining similar data in preterm infants during their first 1–2 weeks of life.

References

1 Blystad W: Blood gas determination on premature infants. III. Investigations on premature infants with recurrent attacks of apnoea. Acta Paediatr Scand 1956;45:211–221.

2 Nelson NM: Members of task force on prolonged apnoea: Reports of the task force on prolonged apnoea of the American Academy of Pediatrics. Pediatrics 1978;61:651–652.

3 Tudehope DI, Rogers YM, Burns YR, Mohay H, O'Callaghan J: Apnoea in very low birthweight infants: Outcome at 2 years. Aust Paediatr J 1986;22:131–134.

4 Daily WJR, Klaus M, Meyer HB: Apnea in premature infants: Monitoring, incidence, heart rate changes, and an effect of environmental temperature. Pediatrics 1969;43:510–518.

5 Alden ER, Mandelkorn R, Woodrum DE, Wennbery RP, Parkes CR, Hodson WA: Morbidity and mortality of infants weighing less than 1000 gms in an intensive care nursery. Pediatrics 1972;50:40–49.

6 Henderson-Smart DJ: The effect of gestational age on the incidence and duration of recurrent apnoea in newborn babies. Aust Paediatr J 1981;17:273–276.

7 Abu-Osba YK, Brouillette RT, Wilson SL, Thach BT: Breathing pattern and transcutaneous oxygen tension during motor activity in preterm infants. Am Rev Respir Dis 1982;125:382–387.

8 Peabody JL, Gregory GA, Willis MM, Philip AGS, Lucey JF: Failure of conventional monitoring to detect apnoea resulting in hypoxaemia. Birth Defects 1979;15:276–284.

9 Southall DP, Bignall S, Stebbens VA, Alexander JR, Rivers RPA, Lissauer T: Pulse oximeter and transcutaneous arterial oxygen measurements in neonatal and paediatric intensive care. Arch Dis Child 1987;62:882–888.

10 Poets CF, Stebbens VA, Alexander JR, Arrowsmith WA, Salfield SAW, Southall DP: Arterial oxygen saturation in preterm infants: Normal values at discharge from the hospital and 6 weeks later. J Pediatr 1992;120:447–454.

11 Stebbens VA, Poets CF, Alexander JA, Arrowsmith WA, Southall DP: Oxygen saturation and breathing patterns in infancy: I. fullterm infants in the second month of life. Arch Dis Child 1991;66:569–573.

12 Groothuis JR, Rosenberg AA: Home oxygen promotes weight gain in infants with bronchopulmonary dysplasia. Am J Dis Child 1987;141:992–995.

13 Teitel D, Sidi, Bernstein D, Heyman MA, Rudolph AM: Chronic hypoxemia in the newborn lamb: cardiovascular, hematopoietic, and growth adaptations. Pediatr Res 1985;19:1004–1010.

14 Rognum TO, Saugstad OD, Øyasæter S, Olaisen B: Elevated levels of hypoxanthine in vitreous humor indicate prolonged cerebral hypoxia in victims of sudden infant death syndrome. Pediatrics 1988;82:615–617.

15 Waggener TB, Frantz ID, Cohlan BA, Stark AR: Mixed and obstructive apneas are related to ventilatory oscillations in premature infants,. J Appl Physiol 1989;66:2818–2826.

16 Upton CJ, Milner AD, Stokes GM: Upper airway patency during apnoea of prematurity. Arch Dis Child 1992;67:419–424.
17 Butcher-Puech MC, Henderson-Smart DJ, Holley D, Lacey JL, Edward DA: Relation between apnoea duration and type and neurological status of preterm infants. Arch Dis Child 1985;60:953–958.
18 Milner AD, Boon AW, Saunders RA, Hopkin IE: Upper airway obstruction and apnoea in preterm babies. Arch Dis Child 1980;55:22–25.
19 Mathew OP: Maintenance of upper airway patency. J Pediatr 1985;106:810–813.
20 Ruggins NR, Milner AD: Site of upper airway obstruction in preterm infants with problematical apnoea. Arch Dis Child 1991;66:787–792.
21 Mathew OP, Roberts JL, Thach BT: Pharyngeal airway obstruction in preterm infants during mixed and obstructive apnea. J Pediatr 1982;100:964–968.
22 Poets CF, Samuels MP, Southall DP: Potential role of intrapulmonary shunting in the genesis of hypoxemic episodes in infants and young children. Pediatrics 1992;90:385–391.
23 Stransky A, Szereda-Przestaszewska M, Widdicombe JG: The effects of lung reflexes on laryngeal resistance and motoneurone discharge. J Physiol 1973;231:417–435.
24 Sant'Ambrogio G: Nervous receptors of the tracheobronchial tree. Ann Rev Physiol 1987;49:611–627.
25 Samuels MP, Poets CF, Stebbens VA, Alexander JR, Southall DP: Oxygen saturation and breathing patterns in preterm infants with cyanotic episodes. Acta Paediatr 1992;81:875–880.
26 Southall DP, Thomas MG, Lambert HP: Severe hypoxaemia in pertussis. Arch Dis Child 1988;63:598–605.
27 Poets CF, Stebbens VA, Alexander JR, Arrowsmith WA, Salfield SAW, Southall DP: Oxygen saturations and breathing patterns in infancy: II. Preterm infants at discharge from special care. Arch Dis Child 1991;66:574–578.
28 Poets CF, Southall DP: Patterns of oxygenation during periodic breathing in preterm infants. Early Hum Dev 1991;26:1–12.
29 Thibeault DW, Wong MM, Auld PAM: Thoracic gas volume changes in premature infants. Pediatrics 1967;60:403–411.
30 Henderson-Smart DJ, Pettigrew AG, Campbell DJ: Clinical apnoea and brain-stem neural function in preterm infants. N Engl J Med 1983;308:353–357.
31 Rigatto H, Brady JB: Periodic breathing and apnea in preterm infants. II. Hypoxia as a primary event. Pediatrics 1972;50:219–227.
32 Fleming PJ, Bryan AC, Bryan MH: Functional immaturity of pulmonary irritant receptors and apnea in newborn preterm infants. Pediatrics 1978;61:515–518.
33 Heldt GP: Development of stability of the respiratory system in preterm infants. J Appl Physiol 1988;65:441–444.
34 Kattwinkel J: Neonatal apnoea: Pathogenesis and therapy. J Pediatr 1977;90:342–347.

Biol Neonate 1994;65:220–230

Jan M. Goplerud
Maria Delivoria-Papadopoulos

Departments of Pediatrics and Physiology, University of Pennsylvania School of Medicine, Philadelphia, Pa., USA

Cerebral Blood Flow and Metabolism during Repeated Asphyxias in Newborn Piglets: Influence of Theophylline

Key Words
Asphyxia
Apnea
Cerebral blood flow
^{31}P NMR
Newborn

Abstract
The effect of theophylline on cerebral blood flow (CBF), oxygen transport, and energy metabolism was investigated during and following brief episodes of asphyxia. CBF was determined by microspheres during control, asphyxia, and recovery with reventilation after a single asphyxia (recovery I) and after 7 repeated asphyxias (recovery II). In addition, cerebral energy metabolism by ^{31}P NMR spectroscopy and cerebral oxygen consumption ($CMRO_2$) in newborn piglets treated with 30 mg/kg theophylline (serum levels 22–25 μg/ml) were compared with nontreated piglets. Theophylline increased $CMRO_2$ during recovery I (348 μmol O_2/min/100 g vs. 144 for non-theophylline) but not during control, asphyxia, or recovery II. There was no significant difference between the theophylline and non-theophylline groups in depletion of phosphoenergetics as measured by ^{31}P NMR.

Introduction

Acute asphyxial events, like apnea, are common in the perinatal period. While the newborn is believed to be relatively more resistant to hypoxemia compared to the adult [1], the extent of the newborn's adaptability to asphyxial stress has yet to be defined. Several recent studies of acute asphyxia produced by disconnecting an anesthetized, paralyzed animal from mechanical ventilation delineate the cerebrovascular perturbations occurring during acute asphyxia [2, 3] and during recovery following asphyxia [3–6]. Although significant redistribution of regional cerebral blood flow results during asphyxia, recovery with reventilation appears to restore cerebrovascular hemodynamics. On a cellular level, however, biochemical disturbances may be occurring altering tissue phosphoenergetics or brain cell membrane function. Furthermore, the cumulative effect of short, but repeated asphyxial events, as may happen in the human newborn with severe apnea is unknown and has important clinical ramifications for future neurological outcome.

In the clinical setting of the intensive care nursery, newborns with recurrent apnea are routinely treated with methylxanthines, including theophylline, aminophylline, and caffeine [7]. All of these act as central neurostimulants which is the rationale for their use in apnea treatment. In addition, theophylline and aminophylline have other actions with

Jan M. Goplerud, MD
Assistant Professor of Pediatrics, Physiology, and Obstetrics/Gynecology
University of Pennsylvania School of Medicine
Hospital of the University of Pennsylvania, 2nd Floor Maloney Building
3400 Spruce Street, Philadelphia, PA 19104 (USA)

possible significance for brain metabolism and the cerebrovasculature. These include functioning as an adenosine antagonist and potentially blocking hypoxia-induced cerebrovasodilation [8, 9] and activity as a phosphodiesterase inhibitor with the capacity to stimulate cellular metabolism via cAMP [10, 11]. While methylxanthines are administered to prevent apnea under the presumption that these individual and repeated asphyxial episodes are harmful, affected infants often continue to have apnea despite therapeutic blood levels of methylxanthine. The present studies were undertaken to test the hypothesis that repeated apneas have cumulative detrimental impact on cerebral cellular phosphoenergetic reserve and that methylxanthines may exacerbate the metabolic impact of these events when they occur. Using a newborn piglet model of acute asphyxia, regional cerebral blood flow measurements with radioactive microspheres were coupled with in vivo ^{31}P NMR spectroscopy of cerebral cortex for continuous monitoring of phosphorous metabolites. Determinations were made before, during, and after repeated asphyxias, both with and without prior administration of methylxanthine (intravenous aminophylline).

Methods

Animal Preparation

Studies were performed on newborn piglets, 3–8 days of age. The piglets were anesthetized with 4% halothane. Following local anesthesia with 2% lidocaine, a tracheostomy was performed and catheters were placed into a femoral artery and vein. For microsphere injection for blood flow measurements, catheters were also positioned in the left atrium, brachial artery, and superior sagittal sinus. In addition, the scalp over the vertex of the brain was reflected to expose the skull for placement of the NMR surface coil, for those piglets undergoing ^{31}P NMR spectroscopy.

Following surgical preparation, the animals were paralyzed (0.5 mg/kg pancuronium bromide) and mechanically ventilated. Halothane was then withdrawn and anesthesia maintained with 70% nitrous oxide and 30% of a compressed air-oxygen mixture sufficient to maintain PaO_2 of 80–110 Torr. No further surgical procedures were performed after halothane was withdrawn and 60–90 min of stabilization was observed before the experiment was begun. Core body temperature was monitored and maintained at 39 °C with a heating pad. Mean arterial blood pressure (MABP), heart rate (HR), and respiratory rate were recorded throughout the study.

Experimental Protocol

Asphyxia was produced in anesthetized, paralyzed, mechanically ventilated newborn piglets by disconnecting from ventilation until bradycardic (heart rate less than 100) – taking approximately 20–90 s from the time ventilation was stopped. Blood flow was determined by microspheres during control, during asphyxia (120–180 s after ventilation stopped), and during recovery with reventilation after a single asphyxia (recovery I) and again during recovery after a seventh of repeated asphyxias (recovery II). The recovery I measurement was made when HR and MABP returned to control levels following the first asphyxia – usually after 4–5 min of reventilation. Over the next 60 min, this asphyxia-recovery cycle was repeated six more times. After a 20- to 30-min recovery from the seventh and final asphyxia, recovery II blood flow measurements were made. Five piglets were studied following theophylline, 30 mg/kg aminophylline given intravenously, with serum theophylline levels of 20–25 μg/ml – while 7 other piglets were in the non-theophylline group. In concurrent experiments, cerebral energy metabolism by ^{31}P NMR spectroscopy and cerebral oxygen consumption ($CMRO_2$) were compared in 4 piglets treated with theophylline and 4 without.

Blood flow measurements were made using 15 μm radioactive microspheres [12]. Microspheres were injected into the left atrial catheter over 15–20 s while a reference withdrawal sample was drawn continuously from a brachial artery. Oxygen transport data were obtained by simultaneous sampling of sagittal sinus blood, representing cerebral venous outflow, and of systemic arterial and venous blood, in conjunction with blood flow determination.

In vivo cerebral magnetic resonance spectroscopy was performed with a 12-inch horizontal bore, 1.9 Tesla spectrometer (Phospho-Energetics, Philadelphia, Pa.). The magnet has a hydrogen frequency of 80.3 MHz, a phosphorus frequency of 32.5 MHz, and a 4-cm diameter, single-turn circular radiofrequency surface coil. During the experiment, the animal is posi-

Table 1. Physiological parameters during blood flow measurements

Newborn piglets	$pH_{(a)}$	$PaCO_2$ mm Hg	PaO_2 mm Hg	MABP mm Hg
Control				
Theophylline	7.42±0.05	37±5	108±27	68±11
Non-theophylline	7.49±0.06	29±2	116±20	72±10
Asphyxia				
Theophylline	7.23±0.13	52±9	24±10	70±18
Non-theophylline	7.27±0.09	54±19	25±5	63±17
Recovery I				
Theophylline	7.39±0.04	34±4	100±16	59±8
Non-theophylline	7.39±0.05	34±6	101±4	77±7
Recovery II				
Theophylline	7.29±0.13	36±6	106±15	61±16
Non-theophylline	7.36±0.18	43±28	96±31	73±3

Physiological parameters: arterial blood gases and MABP during control and experimental conditions during which blood flow and oxygen transport measurements were made. Values represent means ± SD. There are 5 piglets in the theophylline group and 7 piglets in the non-theophylline group.

Table 2. Organ blood flow

Newborn piglets	Control	Asphyxia	Recovery I	Recovery II
Brain				
Theophylline	97±31	94±34	161±71	66±19
Non-theophylline	72±20	70±24	89±37	76±24
Heart				
Theophylline	259±100	605±203	402±154	190±61
Non-theophylline	309±219	572±356	293±144	304±142
Kidneys				
Theophylline	265±59	22±16	186±60	132±49
Non-theophylline	250±65	37±72	207±67	228±102
Skeletal muscle				
Theophylline	29±28	0±0	17±14	15±9
Non-theophylline	17±9	1±3	12±4	11±5

Organ blood flow in ml/min/100 g tissue during control and experimental conditions. Values represent means ± SD. There are 5 piglets in the theophylline group and 7 piglets in the non-theophylline group.

tioned with its brain in the center of the magnetic homogenous field. The surface coil is positioned over the vertex of the intact skull and samples from a region of brain cortex with a 2-cm radius.

Statistical Analysis

Data are reported as means ± SD. Theophylline vs. non-theophylline comparisons were made by paired or unpaired t tests as appropriate. Blood flow and oxygen transport data were analyzed using analysis of variance with repeated measures, followed by Student-Newman-Keuls test where appropriate. Differences were considered significant when $p < 0.05$.

Results

Table 1 represents the blood gas and MABP values during blood flow measurements. Values are expressed as means ± SD. Blood gases are normal during the control, whereas hypoxia, hypercapnia, and acidosis are evident during asphyxia. PaO_2 normalized during both recovery phases, although progressive metabolic acidosis was apparent from recovery I compared to recovery after repeated asphyxias, recovery II. There were no statistically significant differences between the theophylline treated and non-theophylline groups for these parameters.

Figure 1 depicts serum theophylline levels obtained following the 30 mg/kg i.v. aminophylline bolus. By 50–70 min after treatment, serum theophylline levels reached steady state in the 20–25 μg/ml range, remaining at that level throughout the course of the experiment. Theophylline treated piglets had control blood measurements made during this plateau, approximately 90 min after aminophylline was given, while the non-theophylline group was studied a comparable length of time following postsurgical stabilization.

Table 2 presents the organ blood flow to the brain, heart, kidneys, and skeletal muscle for theophylline vs. non-theophylline groups during control and experimental conditions.

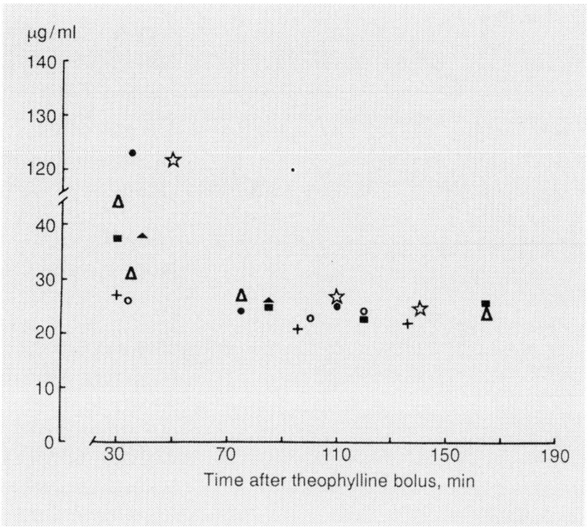

Fig. 1. Serum theophylline levels (μg/ml) in newborn piglets following a 30 mg/kg i.v. bolus dose of aminophylline given at time zero. The symbols represent individual piglets measured sequentially.

Total cerebral blood flow (CBF) was higher in the theophylline group during control, 97 ml/min/100 g (mean ± SD) compared to 72 ml/min/100 g in the non-theophylline piglets. Differences between the theophylline and non-theophylline groups were not statistically significant for any other experimental conditions. During asphyxia, cardiac flow increased while blood flow to the kidneys and skeletal muscle decreased sharply and CBF remained relatively unchanged. With reventilation after asphyxia, blood flow increased to brain, heart, kidneys, and skeletal muscle but without significant theophylline vs. non-theophylline differences.

Regional CBF (rCBF) for theophylline and non-theophylline piglets is given in table 3. Nine brain regions were studied: cerebral gray, cerebral white, caudate, hippocampus, thalamus, midbrain, brain stem, cerebellum, and choroid plexus. While rCBF in the theophylline-treated piglets is consistently higher in each brain region during control compared

Table 3. Regional cerebral blood flow

Newborn piglets	Control	Asphyxia	Recovery I	Recovery II
Cerebral gray				
Theophylline	97 ± 33	68 ± 31	136 ± 79	64 ± 27
Non-theophylline	74 ± 20	55 ± 20	90 ± 35	77 ± 24
Cerebral white				
Theophylline	49 ± 10	42 ± 18	97 ± 58	37 ± 10
Non-theophylline	35 ± 14	32 ± 18	59 ± 54	45 ± 29
Caudate				
Theophylline	87 ± 23	100 ± 42	148 ± 68	68 ± 22
Non-theophylline	72 ± 23	70 ± 34	107 ± 72	88 ± 40
Hippocampus				
Theophylline	58 ± 12*	86 ± 35	123 ± 62	48 ± 14
Non-theophylline	43 ± 12	54 ± 22	62 ± 36	54 ± 22
Thalamus				
Theophylline	100 ± 33	164 ± 66	217 ± 108	77 ± 26
Non-theophylline	79 ± 25	106 ± 40	91 ± 43	78 ± 27
Midbrain				
Theophylline	99 ± 30	196 ± 67*	231 ± 100*	83 ± 24
Non-theophylline	80 ± 27	123 ± 48	101 ± 54	87 ± 30
Brain stem				
Theophylline	88 ± 23	229 ± 49*	211 ± 78*	74 ± 19
Non-theophylline	82 ± 36	134 ± 58	135 ± 130	101 ± 63
Cerebellum				
Theophylline	86 ± 18	105 ± 32	209 ± 103*	68 ± 20
Non-theophylline	70 ± 21	87 ± 36	86 ± 37	75 ± 27
Choroid plexus				
Theophylline	409 ± 196	94 ± 50	305 ± 195	230 ± 101
Non-theophylline	220 ± 106	86 ± 55	183 ± 81	236 ± 106

* $p < 0.05$ for theophylline vs. non-theophylline differences.

Regional cerebral blood flow in ml/min/100 g tissue during control and experimental conditions. Values represent means ± SD. There are 5 piglets in the theophylline group and 7 piglets in the non-theophylline group.

to non-theophylline, only the increase to the hippocampus reached statistical significance. During asphyxia, rCBF redistribution is nonhomogenous with decreased flow to cerebral gray and choroid plexus while flow increase especially to thalamus, midbrain, and brainstem compared to control. Here again theophylline treatment was associated with increased flow compared to non-theophylline with only midbrain and brain stem differences being statistically significant. Blood flow differences in midbrain, brain stem, and cerebellum are seen with theophylline vs. non-theophylline during recovery I.

The oxygen transport data are presented in table 4. Hct values were equivalent for all of

Table 4. Oxygen transport data

Newborn piglets	Cerebral cortical flow ml/min/100 g	O_2 delivery µmol/min/100 g	O_2 extraction $(AO_2 - VO_2)/AO_2$ %	O_2 consumption µmol/min/100 g
Control				
Theophylline	92 ± 34	526 ± 137	36 ± 14	189 ± 49
Non-theophylline	72 ± 20	368 ± 62	51 ± 12	188 ± 32
Asphyxia				
Theophylline	68 ± 31	70 ± 55	60 ± 17	42 ± 33
Non-theophylline	55 ± 20	94 ± 34	64 ± 16	60 ± 22
Recovery I				
Theophylline	136 ± 79	753 ± 242	42 ± 20	316 ± 102*
Non-theophylline	90 ± 35	487 ± 189	30 ± 12	146 ± 57
Recovery II				
Theophylline	64 ± 27	286 ± 67	57 ± 13	163 ± 38
Non-theophylline	77 ± 24	409 ± 127	55 ± 16	225 ± 70

* $p < 0.05$ for theophylline vs. non-theophylline differences.

Oxygen transport data based on systemic arterial-sagittal sinus oxygen differences during control and experimental conditions. Values represent means ± SD. There are 5 piglets in the theophylline group and 7 piglets in the non-theophylline group.

the conditions at 30 ± 3%. The cerebral cortical oxygen delivery and consumption were determined from systemic arterial-sagittal sinus differences for control, asphyxia, recovery I, and recovery II. There were no significant differences in oxygen consumption between the theophylline-treated and non-theophylline groups during control or during asphyxia, although oxygen delivery was greater for the theophylline group because of the higher cortical flow. However, during recovery I the theophylline group had significantly higher oxygen consumption compared to non-theophylline. This difference was not present during recovery II after 6 additional episodes of asphyxia-reventilation.

Representative ^{31}P NMR spectra obtained during the various conditions of the experimental protocol are illustrated in figure 2. The first spectrum in the upper left, labelled 'control', is a typical normal NMR spectrum of the newborn piglet. Identified are the 7 phosphorus compound peaks characteristic of the newborn. There are distinctive peaks caused by each of the three phosphate groups of ATP (alpha, beta, and gamma); the phosphocreatine peak occurs at 0 ppm. The inorganic phosphorous peak, P_i, is located to its left and is low in normal or control state. The other two labelled peaks are PME, attributed to phosphorylated monoesters, and the PDE peak, representing phosphodiesters. In the subsequent spectra, only the P_i and PCr peaks are labelled. The second proceeding from the left was taken during the first asphyxia – here called apnea – and shows an increase in P_i while PCr has fallen. The middle spectrum represents recovery from asphyxia 1 and PCr has increased while P_i is diminished. The next spectrum is from asphyxia 6 and again PCr is

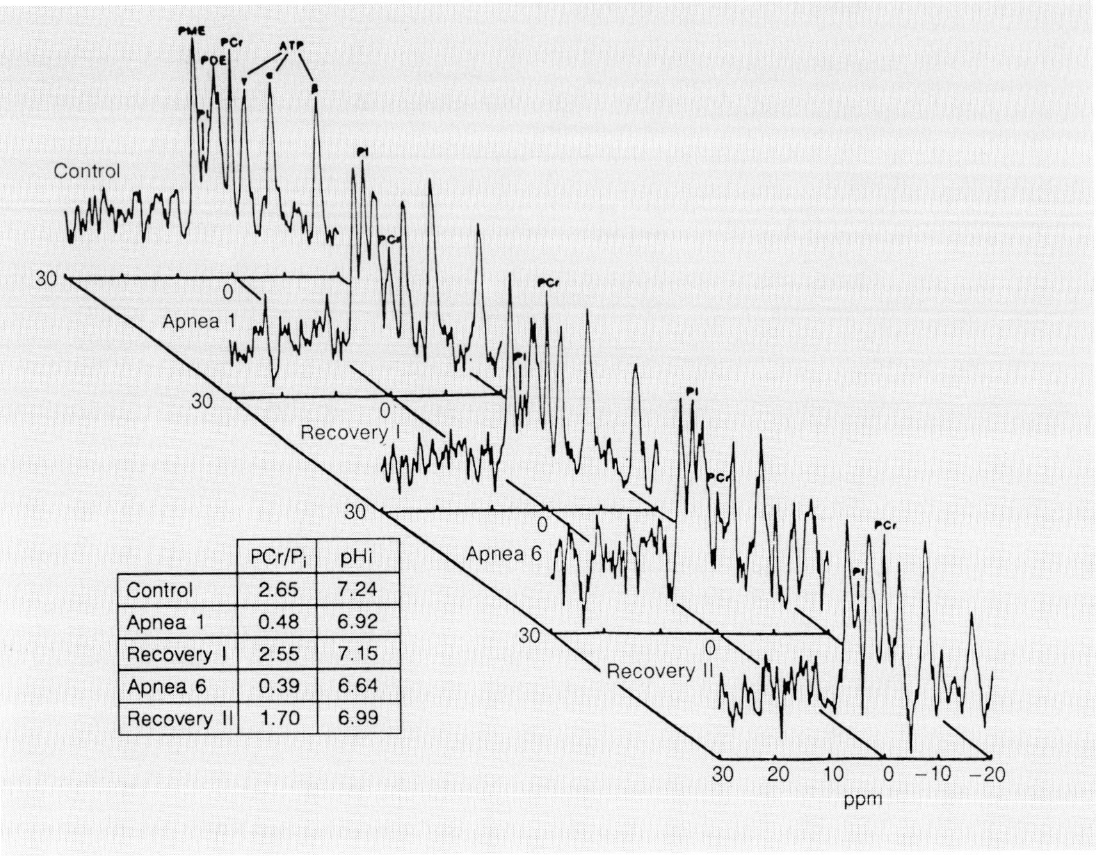

	PCr/P$_i$	pHi
Control	2.65	7.24
Apnea 1	0.48	6.92
Recovery I	2.55	7.15
Apnea 6	0.39	6.64
Recovery II	1.70	6.99

Fig. 2. ^{31}P NMR spectra representing individual events in the course of a single experiment. Labelled peaks are phosphomonoester (PME), inorganic phosphate (P_i), phosphodiester (PDE), phosphocreatine (PCr), and alpha, beta, and gamma peaks of adenosine triphosphate (ATP). The term apnea is used for the episodes of acute asphyxia.

low while P_i is high. Finally, during recovery II, PCr has been restored and Pi_i, although lower than during asphyxia, is still higher than control.

The two peaks of greatest importance in the cerebral phosphoenergetic studies are the PCr and P_i peaks. Since absolute quantitation is difficult with in vivo magnetic resonance spectroscopy, spectra are analyzed by measuring the height of a given peak from baseline. The relative amounts of phosphocreatine and inorganic phosphorus are then expressed as a ratio of peak heights known as the PCr/P_i. Intracellular pH, or pHi, is calculated from the chemical shift of the P_i peak with respect to the PCr. The table accompanying figure 2 shows the PCr/P_i and pHi values corresponding to each of the 5 spectra.

Figure 3 demonstrates the PCr/P_i and pHi values during repeated asphyxias. The horizontal axis is time in minutes. Intracellular pH values are plotted in the upper graph while the lower graph depicts PCr/P_i values. Arrows indicate the times at which ventilation is

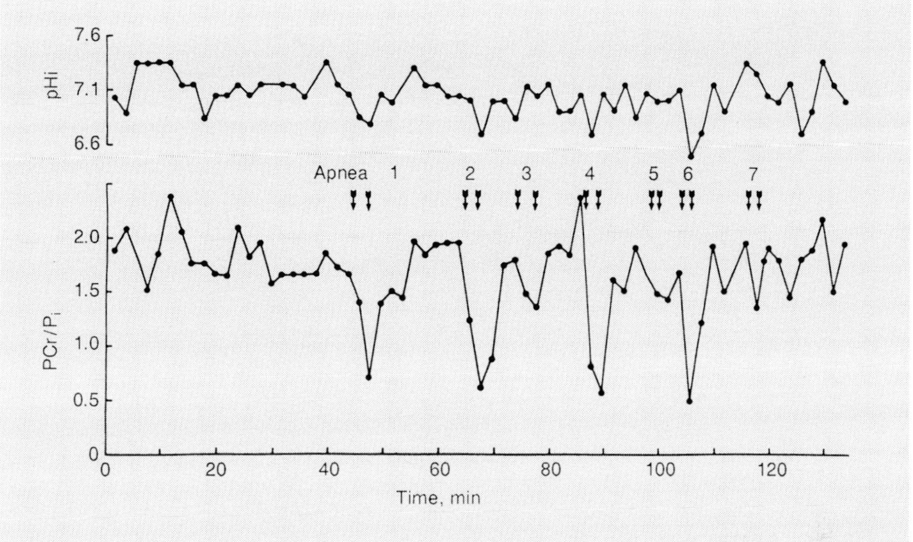

Fig. 3. ^{31}P NMR spectroscopy data from a representative experiment of the non-theophylline group. PCr/P_i ratio and intracellular pH (pHi) are graphed against time in minutes with arrows indicating the times at which mechanical ventilation was stopped and restarted for each apnea.

stopped and resumed for each of 7 asphyxia episodes in a representative study. There is a very rapid and dramatic fall in PCr/P_i in response to each asphyxia with a corresponding fall in pHi. While PCr/P_i is quickly restored after each successive asphyxia, pHi recovers more slowly and the gradual decline in the overall level of pHi suggests a cumulative effect of the repeated apneas.

Representative graphs of ^{31}P NMR spectroscopy data for a theophylline-treated piglet and a non-theophylline piglet are depicted for comparison in figure 4. While there is considerable variability in the PCr/P_i range between piglets and from asphyxia to asphyxia, the recovery of PCr/P_i with reventilation after asphyxias was generally higher in the theophylline-treated group consistent with the higher $CMRO_2$ during recovery I. However, because of the variability in baseline PCr/P_i between piglets, it was not possible to determine the significance of this observed difference. Similarly, pHi was not significantly different between groups over the course of repeated asphyxias.

Discussion

The present studies combine CBF measurements by microspheres, oxygen transport determinations, and continuous in vivo ^{31}P NMR spectroscopy to analyze and integrate hemodynamic and brain cellular phosphoenergetic consequences of single and repeated acute asphyxial insults in newborn piglets, both with and without theophylline. Because these studies investigate brain cellular metabolic response to asphyxia, a theophylline dose likely to inhibit phosphodiesterase, and thus increase cAMP, was chosen, theophylline doses of 6 [13] and 10 mg/kg [14] had pre-

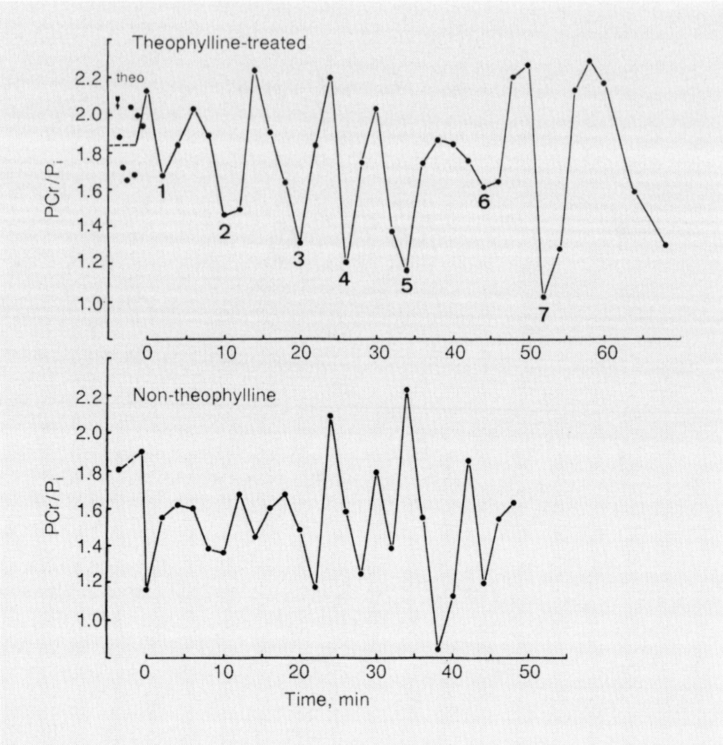

Fig. 4. Comparison of 31P NMR spectroscopy data for representative experiments of a theophylline-treated and a non-theophylline treated piglet. PCr/P_i ratio is plotted against time in minutes with the sequential episodes of asphyxia numbered.

viously been shown not to alter CBF or $CMRO_2$ in newborn piglets. However, a theophylline dose of 25 mg/kg or higher had been found to increase cAMP and cGMP levels in rat brain [11]. Using intravenous aminophylline at a dose of 30 mg/kg – the equivalent of 25 mg/kg theophylline –, we obtained serum theophylline levels consistent with earlier pharmacokinetic studies in newborn piglets [15], achieving steady state levels an hour after intravenous administration.

We have previously characterized the nonhomogenous rCBF during acute asphyxia in the newborn piglet [3]. Blood flow to the cerebral cortex and choroid plexus decreased while increases were seen in other brain regions, particularly the thalamus, midbrain, and brain stem. During recovery with reventilation, following a single and after repeated asphyxias, CBF distribution was more uniform. Studies in other newborn species have corroborated our CBF findings during asphyxia [2] and during recovery [4, 5] using the same model of asphyxia, although none of these studies examined both the asphyxia and postasphyxial phase in the same animal. While the nonhomogeneous rCBF was present in the current study in both our theophylline and non-theophylline groups, the theophylline group had significantly greater rCBF increases to midbrain and brain stem during asphyxia and recovery I compared to non-theophylline. In addition, the cerebellum in the theophylline-treated group had significantly higher CBF during recovery I compared to non-theophylline. These results are consistent with theophylline's role as a phosphodiesterase inhibitor, thus increasing tissue levels of cAMP particularly in those brain regions known to be most metabolically active. However, theophylline does not appear to block cerebral vasodilation during asphyxia or in the acute recovery after asphyxia as might be expected by adenosine antagonism. Adenosine has been shown to have a role in regulating cerebral hyperemia during hypoxic hypoxia in the newborn [9]. Theophylline's influence on cerebrovascular response may be dose-dependent [8] with its phosphodiesterase inhibition prevailing at the dose used in the current studies. When the effect of methylxanthines on cerebral blood flow velocity (CBFV) has been studied in preterm infants, results have been variable at clinically therapeutic doses of 5–10 mg/kg [16–19]. Doppler ultrasound CBFV was reduced in one report [16] and unchanged in another [17] after intravenous aminophylline, while xenon-133 clearance measurement of CBF showed a 13.8% reduction in CBF after aminophylline [18] but unaltered visual evoked response as a measure of cerebral function. Similarly, CBF based on near infrared spectroscopy (NIRS) determinations was reduced 29% by intravenous aminophylline [19].

We found no significant differences in $CMRO_2$ between the theophylline-treated and non-theophylline groups during control or during asphyxia, although oxygen delivery was greater for the theophylline group because of the higher cortical flow. However, during recovery I the theophylline group had significantly higher $CMRO_2$ compared to non-theophylline. This may reflect compensation for a higher oxygen debt acquired during asphyxia or possibly a theophylline-stimulated increase in metabolism during the recovery-hyperemia phase with reventilation. This finding of increased postasphyxial $CMRO_2$ in the theophylline-treated brain led us to hypothesize that repeated episodes of asphyxia-recovery at this increased metabolic rate might more quickly deplete tissue energy stores. Thus, theophylline could have a deleterious effect on the brain's capacity to withstand repetitive asphyxial events. The theophylline-associated increase in $CMRO_2$ did not persist in recovery II, after six additional asphyxia-reventilation episodes. In fact, $CMRO_2$ in the theophylline group was lower during recovery II compared to non-theophylline, although the difference was not statistically significant. This could represent a depletion of brain tissue energy reserve. We have previously investigated the effect of single and repeated apneas on brain cortical Na^+,K^+-ATPase activity and lipid peroxidation in newborn piglets [20]. As a membrane-bound enzyme central to brain cell membrane function, Na^+,K^+-ATPase was significantly inhibited after single and repeated asphyxias, associated with an accumulation of lipid peroxidation products. Since Na^+,K^+-ATPase activity accounts for 40–60% of the brain's energy use [21] its inhibition could account for decreased brain $CMRO_2$. Depression of cellular respiration has been reported after repeated hypoxic episodes in human newborns [22] studied with noninvasive infrared monitoring of cerebral oxygenation. When hypoxic episodes came in series or were prolonged, cytochrome a+a3 reduction, which occurred simultaneously with hemoglobin deoxygenation, lagged behind hemoglobin oxygenation during recovery.

In the current studies we used ^{31}P NMR spectroscopy to compare the cerebral cortical phosphoenergetic response of theophylline-treated and non-theophylline groups to repeated episodes of asphyxia-reventilation. While both groups had marked fluctuations in PCr/P_i and pHi, as depicted in figures 3 and 4, in response to sequential asphyxias, animal-to-animal variability precluded assessment of significant differences between the groups.

Conclusions

In conclusion, in the present studies in newborn piglets, theophylline did not appear to interfere with cerebrovascular dilation to either asphyxia or recovery as might be predicted by its potential to block adenosine. Instead, theophylline consistently increased cerebral blood flow with the most significant increase to midbrain and brain stem regions, consistent with their greater metabolic activity and possibly due to inhibition of phosphodiesterase. Finally, as measured by ^{31}P NMR spectroscopy, cerebral cortical phosphoenergetic reserves were not depleted by repeated episodes of asphyxia despite a theophylline-stimulated increase in O_2 consumption during recovery.

Acknowledgements

Supported in part by NIH Physiology Research Training Grant 5T32HL07027-10 and NIH HD-20337. We thank Dr. Leslie Shaw for the measurement of theophylline levels and we sincerely appreciate the secretarial assistance of Dorothy Zurlo in the preparation of this manuscript.

References

1 Vannuci RC, Duffy TE: Cerebral metabolism in newborn dogs during reversible asphyxia. Ann Neurol 1977;1:528–534.
2 Hernandez MJ, Hawkins RA, Brennan RW: Regional cerebral blood flow during neonatal asphyxia; in Passoneau JV, Hawkins RA, Lust WD, Welsh FA (eds): Cerebral Metabolism and Neural Function. Baltimore, Williams & Wilkins, 1980, pp 196–201.
3 Goplerud JM, Wagerle LC, Delivoria-Papadopoulos M: Regional cerebral blood flow response during and after acute asphyxia in newborn piglets. J Appl Physiol 1989;66:2827–2832.
4 McPhee AJ, Kotagal UR, Kleinman LI: Cerebrovascular hemodynamics during and after recovery from acute asphyxia in the newborn dog. Pediatr Res 1985;19:645.
5 Rosenberg AA: Cerebral blood flow and O_2 metabolism after asphyxia in neonatal lambs. Pediatr Res 1986; 20:778–782.
6 Stonestreet BS, Laptook A, Schanler R, Oh W: Hemodynamic responses to asphyxia in spontaneously breathing newborn term and premature lambs. Early Human Dev 1982; 7:81–97.
7 Aranda JV, Turman T: Methylxanthines in apnea of prematurity. Clin Perinatol 1979;6:87–108.
8 Hoffman WE, Albrecht RF, Miletich DJ: The role of adenosine in CBF increases during hypoxia in young vs. aged rats. Stroke 1984;15: 124–129.
9 Laudignon N, Farri E, Beharry K, Rex J, Aranda JV: Influence of adenosine on cerebral blood flow during hypoxic hypoxia in the newborn piglet. J Appl Physiol 1990;68: 1534–1541.
10 Holowach-Thurston J, Hauhart RE, Dirgo JA: Aminophylline increases cerebral metabolic rate and decreases anoxic survival in young mice. Science 1978;201:649–651.
11 Stefanovich V: Influence of theophylline on concentrations of cyclic 3′,5′-adenosine monophosphate and cyclic 3′,5′-guanosine monophosphate of rat brain. Neurochem Res 1979;4:587–594.
12 Heymann MA, Payne BD, Hoffman JIE, Rudolph AM: Blood measurements with radionuclide-labeled particles. Prog Cardiovasc Dis 1977; 20:55–59.
13 Stonestreet BS, Nowicki PT, Hansen NB, Petit R, Oh W: Effect of aminophylline on brain blood flow in the newborn piglet. Dev Pharmacol Ther 1983;6:248–258.
14 McPhee AJ, Maxwell GM: The effect of theophylline on regional cerebral blood flow responses to hypoxia in newborn piglets. Pediatr Res 1987;21:573–578.
15 Kearns GL, Hill DE, Tumbelson ME: Theophylline and caffeine disposition in the neonatal piglet. Dev Pharmacol Ther 1986;9:389–401.
16 Rosenkrantz ES, Oh W: Aminophylline reduces cerebral blood flow velocity in low birthweight infants. Am J Dis Child 1984;138:489–491.
17 Ghai V, Raju TNK, Kim SY, McCulloch KM: Regional cerebral blood flow velocity after aminophylline therapy in premature newborn infants. J Pediatr 1989;114:870–873.
18 Pryds O, Schneider S: Aminophylline reduces cerebral blood flow in stable, preterm infants without affecting the visual evoked potential. Eur J Pediatr 1991;150:366–369.
19 McDonnell M, Ives WK, Hope PL: Intravenous aminophylline and cerebral blood flow in preterm infants. Arch Dis Child 1992;67:416–418.
20 Goplerud JM, Mishra OP, Delivoria-Papadopoulos M: Brain cell membrane dysfunction following actue asphyxia in newborn piglets. Biol Neonate 1992;61:33–41.
21 Astrup J, Sorensen PM, Sorensen HR: Oxygen and glucose consumption related to Na^+-K^+ transport in canine brain. Stroke 1981;12:720–726.
22 Brazy JE, Lewis DV, Jobsis FF: Noninvasive monitoring of cerebral oxygenation in preterm infants: Preliminary observations. Pediatrics 1985;75:217–225.

Biol Neonate 1994;65:231–234

Cl. Gaultier

Laboratoire de Physiologie,
INSERM CJF 8909,
Hôpital A.-Beclere,
Clamart, France

Apnea and Sleep State in Newborns and Infants

Key Words
Active sleep
Hyperthermia
Sleep deprivation
Meperidine
Obstructive apnea
Periodic breathing
REM sleep

Abstract
Many studies have shown a greater frequency of apneas in active sleep than in quiet sleep in healthy newborns and infants, both full-term and preterm. The ontogeny of increased apnea during active sleep is related to phasic inhibitory-excitatory central mechanisms occurring during active sleep. Respiratory instability in active sleep can be increased by factors which modify the newborn's or infant's homeostasis. We have shown: (1) an increase in body temperature (0.8 °C) significantly augments periodic breathing in preterm infants at 40 weeks postconceptional age; (2) maternal administration of meperidine is followed by a significant increase in number of apneas during the first hours of life in full-term newborns, but only during active sleep; (3) sleep deprivation induces significantly more obstructive respiratory events in active sleep than in quiet sleep in infants. Active sleep appears to be a risk period for exaggeration of the occurrence of apneas when the newborn's or infant's homeostasis is disturbed.

This short review has two aims: (1) to summarize current knowledge of the relationship between apnea and sleep state during the early period of life, and (2) to consider the potential vulnerability of active sleep as compared to quiet sleep when the infant's homeostasis is disturbed.

Over the last two decades, many studies have shown that apneas of short duration are common during the early period of life [1–5]. Apneas are mostly central [2]. Apneas are more frequent in preterm than in full-term newborns [3]. Apnea frequency decreases with postconceptional age [1–3]. In full-term infants at 1 week of age, the obstructive apnea index is very low compared to the central apnea index and decreases further with advancing postnatal age. Some studies on apneas during the early period of life have focused on the role of sleep state in relation to apnea occurrence. In all studies except one [6], apnea was more frequent in active sleep (AS) than in quiet sleep (QS) in preterm or fullterm newborns [1–3, 5]. Lee et al. [6] recently reported that the higher frequency of apneas in AS appears only after 44 weeks postconceptional age.

The higher frequency of apneas in AS during the early period of life is in contrast to what happens later on in children and adolescents, in whom few apneas occur, especially during stage 1–2 NREM sleep [7, 8]. Potential mechanisms for the greater respiratory instability in AS than in QS during the early period of life include the association of overall immaturity of the brain stem centers and the respi-

Cl. Gaultier
Laboratoire de Physiologie
INSERM CJF 8909
Hôpital A.-Beclere
F–92141 Clamart (France)

0006–3126/94/
0654–0231$5.00/0

ratory pump, and phasic inhibitory-excitatory mechanisms inherent to active sleep.

Rhythmic activity must be maintained through continuous postsynaptic excitation. Neuronal immaturity may be a major factor responsible for repetitive apneas in the early period of life. Neuronal immaturity is characterized by a lack of dendritic arborization, few synaptic connections and insufficient excitatory drive. As a result, mechanisms implicated in establishing rhythmic respiration are immature. Immaturity influences both respiratory pattern generation and other brain stem activity. Henderson-Smart et al. [9] have shown that preterm infants with numerous apneas have prolonged latency responses to brain stem auditory-evoked potentials compared to infants of similar gestational age with few apneas, suggesting that the occurrence of apneas is correlated with immature neural function in the brain stem.

Schulte et al. [10] have shown that in preterm infants, apneic spells predominantly occur during the periods of decreased spinal motoneurone excitability during active sleep. Frequent apneas during the early period of life in active sleep may be an exaggeration of the normally phasic inhibitory-excitatory central mechanisms occurring during this sleep state. Irregular phasic respiratory patterns of REM sleep occur in synchrony with other brain stem phasic activity, such as rapid eye movements. In infants at 1 month of age, Haddad et al. [11] showed that tidal volume and the total duration of the respiratory cycle decrease with increasing frequency of rapid eye movements. Inhibitory mechanisms during REM sleep affect muscles involved in respiratory adaptation, i.e. upper airway muscles and intercostal muscles. Upper airway muscle inhibition may make upper airway obstruction more likely to occur. This has been implicated as an important contributory factor in prolonging apneic events [12]. Inhibition of the intercostal muscles affect the stability of the chest wall in AS in the early period of life because of the immaturity of the respiratory pump.

The main characteristic of the immaturity of the respiratory pump is a high chest wall compliance relative to lung compliance [13]. The highly compliant chest wall of the newborn is subject to inward motion when intercostal muscles are inhibited in AS. Preterm and full-term infants spend nearly 100% of AS time with thoracic paradox. Thoracic paradox during inspiration has been shown to be associated with mechanical disturbances: (1) decrease in end expiratory lung volume [14, 15] which decreases lung O_2 stores; (2) decrease in transcutaneous PO_2 [16]; (3) increase in the diaphragmatic work of breathing [17], and (4) inhibitory intercostal-phrenic reflex [18]. All these disturbances may favor occurrence of apneas. However, their role is arguable, since the frequency of apneas decreases in preterm infants between 31 and 40 weeks postconceptional age whereas the time spent in thoracic paradox in AS does not change [3].

Finally, ventilatory responses to chemical stimuli are lower in AS than in QS. Rigatto et al. [19] have documented a lower ventilatory response to hypoxia in AS compared to QS in preterm infants. Three studies have reported a lower ventilatory response to hypercapnia in AS and proposed three mechanisms: loss of rib cage contribution to ventilation [20], decrease in diaphragmatic EMG activity [21, 22] and inhibition of abdominal muscle activity that contributes to ventilatory responses in QS [22]. Lower ventilatory responses to chemical stimuli in AS may favor more frequent and longer apneas.

Many factors can enhance respiratory instability during the early period of life [23]. Among them are metabolic disorders, neurologic disorders, hypoxia, viral infection, hyperthermia, sleep deprivation, and drug administration. We hypothesized that AS should be more vulnerable than QS to disturbances in infant's homeostasis, and conducted three studies to compare the effects of hyperthermia, sleep deprivation and drug administration on breathing pattern in AS and QS in healthy newborns and infants.

In healthy preterm newborns at a mean postconceptional age of 40 weeks, we measured the effect of a mild increase in body temperature (0.8 °C) [24]. Hyperthermia did not modify sleep organization. Increase in body temperature was responsible for a significant increase in the time spent in periodic breathing with or without apneic oscillations but only in AS. Several potential mechanisms may explain the increased respiratory instability observed during hyperthermia in AS. Periodicity occurs as a result of relative lack of damping provided by O_2 stores and it has been shown that the end expiratory lung volume decreases in AS [14, 15]. Additionally, periodicity may result from an increase in metabolic response. More active metabolic responses to thermal stress have been shown in AS in human newborns [25].

We have also reported the effect of sleep deprivation in healthy infants at 3 months of age [26]. They were studied during afternoon naps on a baseline day and on the following day after 4 hours sleep deprivation. Sleep deprivation was not followed by AS rebound. Sleep deprivation induced a significant increase in periodic breathing but only in AS. Additionally, sleep deprivation resulted in a significant increase in obstructive respiratory events, especially in AS. The enhancement of periodic breathing in AS may be related to the demonstrated depression of ventilatory responses to chemical stimuli after sleep deprivation [27]. These ventilatory responses are normally lower in AS than in QS. Decrease in genioglossal EMG activity is commonly described in AS, and sleep deprivation selectively decreases genioglossal EMG activity [28]. Consequently, it may be understood why obstructive respiratory events occur preferentially in AS after sleep deprivation.

Meperidine is the drug most widely used to control labor pain. The risks of neonatal depression in newborns with a low Apgar score at birth whose mothers received meperidine have been recognized for a long time. We considered whether newborns with a normal Apgar score have abnormal breathing patterns during the first hour of life consequent to maternal meperidine administration, and hypothesized that if present, the effect of meperidine should be prominent in AS [29]. We compared a group of full-term newborns whose mothers received meperidine to a control group during the first 6 h of life. Meperidine did not modify the wake-sleep pattern in those newborns compared to control infants. Meperidine significantly increased the number and duration of apneas, and the time spent with an O_2 saturation (SaO_2) less than 90%, but only in AS. Meperidine has been shown to induce depression of ventilatory responses to chemical stimuli in awake adults [30]. We speculated that the depression of the normally decreased ventilatory responses to chemical stimuli, associated with a longer time spent with $SaO_2 < 90\%$, may explain the increase in apnea number and duration, in AS.

In summary, the higher frequency of apneas in AS compared to QS during the early period of life may be an exaggeration of the normally phasic inhibitory-excitatory central mechanisms occurring in AS because of immaturity of the brain stem centers and the respiratory pump. When the infant's homeostasis is disturbed, AS appears to be more vulnerable for increasing respiratory instability than QS. This greater vulnerability of AS is of clinical relevance since AS occupies a large proportion of sleep time during the early period of life.

References

1 Hoppenbrouwers T, Hodgman JE, Harper RM, Hofman E, Sterman MB, McGinty DJ: Polygraphic studies of normal infants during the first six months of life. III. Incidence of apnea and periodic breathing. Pediatrics 1977;60:418–425.

2 Guilleminault C, Ariagno R, Korobkin R, Nagel L, Baldwin R, Coons S, Owem M: Mixed and obstructive sleep apnea and near miss for sudden infant death syndrome 2. Comparison of near miss and normal control infants by age. Pediatrics 1979;64:882–891.

3 Curzi-Dascalova L, Christova-Guerguieva E: Respiratory pauses in normal prematurely born infants. Biol Neonate 1983;44:325–332.

4 Gould JB, Lee AFS, James O, Sander L, Teager H, Fineberg N: The sleep state characteristics of apnea during infancy. Pediatrics 1977;59:182–194.

5 Gabriel M, Albani M, Schulte FJ: Apneic spells and sleep states in preterm infants. Pediatrics 1976;57:142–147.

6 Lee D, Caces R, Kwiatkowski K, Cates D, Rigatto H: A developmental study on types and frequency distribution of short apneas (3 to 15 seconds) in term and preterm infants. Pediatr Res 1987;22:344–349.

7 Carskadon MA, Harvey K, Dement WC, Guilleminault C, Simmons FB, Anders TF: Respiration during sleep in children. West J Med 1978;128:477–481.

8 Tabachnik E, Muller NL, Bryan AC, Levison H: Changes in ventilation and chest wall mechanics during sleep in normal adolescents. J Appl Physiol 1981;51:557–564.

9 Henderson-Smart DJ, Pettigrew AG, Campbell DJ: Clinical apnea and brainstem neural function in preterm infants. N Engl J Med 1983;308:353–357.

10 Schulte FJ, Busse C, Eichorn W: Rapid eye movement sleep, motoneurone inhibition, and apneic spells in preterm infants. Pediatr Res 1977;11:709–713.

11 Haddad GG, Lai TL, Mellins RB: Determination of ventilatory pattern in REM sleep in normal infants. J Appl Physiol 1982;53:52–56.

12 Thach BT, Stark AR: Spontaneous neck flexion and airway obstruction during apneic spells in preterm infants. J Pediatr 1979;94:275–281.

13 Bryan AC, Gaultier C: The thorax in children; in Macklem PT, Roussos H (eds): The Thorax, part B. New York, Marcel Dekker, 1985, pp 871–888.

14 Henderson-Smart DJ, Read DJC: Reduced lung volume during behavioral active sleep in newborn. J Appl Physiol 1979;46:1081–1085.

15 Walti H, Moriette G, Radvanyi-Bouvet MF, Chaussain M, Morel-Kahn F, Pajot N, Relier JP: Influence of breathing pattern on functional residual capacity in sleeping newborn infants. J Dev Physiol 1986;8:167–172.

16 Martin RJ, Okken A, Rubin D: Arterial oxygen tension during active and quiet sleep. J Pediatr 1979;94:271–274.

17 Guslits BG, Gaston SE, Bryan MY, England SJ, Bryan AC: Diaphragmatic work of breathing in premature human infants. J Appl Physiol 1987;62:1410–1415.

18 Hagan R, Bryan AC, Bryan MH, Gulston G: Neonatal chest wall afferents and regulation of respiration. J Appl Physiol 1977;42:362–367.

19 Rigatto H, Kalapesi Z, Leahy FN, Durand M, McCallum M, Cates D: Ventilatory response to 100% and 15% O_2 during wakefulness and sleep in preterm infants. Early Hum Dev 1982;7:1–10.

20 Honma Y, Wilkes D, Bryan MH, Bryan AC: Rib cage and abdominal contributions to ventilatory response to CO_2 in infants. J Appl Physiol 1984;56:1211–1216.

21 Moriette G, van Reempts P, Moore M, Cates D, Rigatto H: The effect of rebreathing CO_2 on ventilation and diaphragmatic electromyography in newborns infants. Respir Physiol 1985;62:387–397.

22 Praud JP, Egreteau L, Benlabed M, Curzi-Dascalova L, Nedelcoux H, Gaultier Cl: Abdominal muscle activity during CO_2 rebreathing in sleeping neonates. J Appl Physiol 1991;70:1344–1350.

23 Gaultier C: Respiratory adaptation during sleep in infants. Lung 1990;167(suppl):905–911.

24 Berterottiere D, D'Allest AM, Dehan M, Gaultier C: Effects of increase in body temperature on the breathing pattern in premature infants. J Dev Physiol 1990;13:303–308.

25 Fleming PJ, Levine MR, Azaz Y, Johnson P: The effect of sleep state on the metabolic response to cold stress in newborn infants; in Jones CT (ed): Fetal and Neonatal Development. Ithaca, Perinatology Press, 1988, pp 643–647.

26 Canet E, Gaultier Cl, D'Allest AM, Dehan M: Effects of sleep deprivation on respiratory events during sleep in healthy infants. J Appl Physiol 1989;66:1158–1163.

27 Schiffman PL, Trontell MC, Mazar MF, Edelman NH: Sleep deprivation decreases ventilatory response to CO_2 but not load compensation. Chest 1983;84:695–698.

28 Leiter JC, Knuth SL, Bartlett D: The effect of sleep deprivation on activity of the genioglossus muscle. Am Rev Respir Dis 1985;132:1242–1245.

29 Hamza J, Benlabed M, Orhant E, Escourrou P, Curzi-Dascalova L, Gaultier Cl: Neonatal pattern of breathing during active and quiet sleep after maternal administration of meperidine. Pediatr Res 1992;32:412–416.

30 Kryger MH, Yacoub O, Dosman J, Macklem PT, Anthonisen NR: Effect of meperidine on occlusion pressure response to hypercapnia and hypoxia with and without external inspiratory resistance. Am Rev Respir Dis 1976;114:333–340.

Biol Neonate 1994;65:235–239

Mechanisms of Obstructive Sleep Apneas in Infants

A. Kahn[a]
J. Groswasser[a]
M. Sottiaux[a]
E. Rebuffat[b]
P. Franco[c]

[a] Pediatric Sleep Unit, University Children's Hospital,
[b] Free University of Brussels,
[c] University Clinic Erasme, Brussels, Belgium

Abstract

During sleep, infants with obstructive sleep apneas are characterised by snoring, laborious breathing, and profuse sweating. During wakefulness, they may have breath-holding spells, and during feeding, difficult breathing and swallowing coordination. Abnormal weight, difficult growth, and recurring ear infections may also develop. During sleep apneas, cinefluoroscopy shows approximation of tongue and hypopharyngeal tissues, with an obliteration of the air space. The obstructed breaths occur mainly in REM, and light NREM sleep, associated with total short sleep time, and frequent arousals. Preterm infants, and term neonates are more prone to obstructive apneas than older healthy infants. Apneas are more frequently seen in boys and in case of excess in body weight. Obstructive apneas are frequently associated with upper airway anatomic abnormalities: malformations, soft tissue infiltration, and neurologic lesions impairing muscle contractions. Alterations of the autonomic nervous control may induce airways obstructions. Contributing factors include mucopolysaccharide storage disease, hypothyroidism, or Down's syndrome. Superimposed factors may occur, such as nasal obstruction, secretions in the airways, or tissue edema. Pressure- and chemo-sensitive reflexes may also favor obstruction. Environmental factors also contribute to the development of sleep apneas: body position, neck flexion, sleep deprivation, or the effects of sedative drugs.

Key Words
Apneas
Obstructive apneas
Sleep
Infants
Sudden infant death syndrome
Autonomic nervous system
Breath-holding spells
Polysomnography
Allergy
Death

Introduction

The present review focusses on obstructive events of the upper airways that occur during sleep in infants between 1 and 6 months of age. We do not address other forms of airways obstructions, such as smothering, accidental suffocation, or major respiratory infections.

A. Kahn
Pediatric Sleep Unit
University Children's Hospital Reine Fabiola
Avenue J.J.-Crocq 15
B–1020 Brussels (Belgium)

0006–3126/94/
0654–0235$5.00/0

Table 1. Major osteomuscular factors related to obstructive apneas

Facial dysmorphia
Micrognathia
Pierre-Robin Syndrome
Arthrogryposis
Temporomandibular joint ankylosis
Facial abnormalities
Crouzon disease
Larsen syndrome
Trisomy 21 (Down's syndrome)
Traecher-Collin syndrome
Fronto-metaphyseal displagia
Nasal septal defect
Neuromuscular disorders
Cerebral palsy
Acquired dysautonomia
Chiari malformation
Syringomyelo-bulbia
Congenital myopathy
Myotonic dystrophy

Presentation of Sleep Apneas

Infants with obstructed breathing events are characterised during sleep by heavy and laborious breathing, snoring, and profuse night sweats. During wakefulness, they may show breath-holding spells, and distress during feeding. Abnormal weight, delayed growth, and recurring ear infections may also develop [1, 2].

Cinefluoroscopic findings show that the tongue and hypopharyngeal soft tissues are closing up during an apneic episode, obliterating the air space [3, 4]. The obstruction of air flow are confirmed by polysomnographic recordings, showing flat tracings from the nasal and oral thermistors, despite continuous deflections from thoracic strain gauges [5, 6]. These obstructive apneas occur mainly in REM and light NREM sleep. They are associated with shorter total sleep time, and frequent short arousals [6].

Factors Associated with Sleep Apneas

Several studies have shown that obstructive and mixed sleep apneas are rare in healthy infants [6–8]. Factors related to the development of obstructive apneas are the child's age, sex, and weight. Obstructive and mixed apneas are more frequently seen in premature than in full-term infants [9]. They are also more frequent in boys than in girls [5, 6]. The cause for the sex-related difference in apnea frequency is not known. Excessive body weight in otherwise healthy infants may also favor obstructive sleep apneas [10] (table 1).

Some authors consider obstructive sleep apneas in infants to be most frequently associated with an upper airway *anatomic abnormality*. Such anatomic problems that reduce the patency of the airways may be divided into three major groups: bone malformations, soft tissue infiltration, and neurologic lesions impairing muscle contractions [1, 2, 6, 11]. Causes frequently reported include craniofacial abnormalities, micrognathia, cleft palate, long soft palate, adenotonsillar hypertrophy, laryngomalacia, supraglottic edema, subglottic stenosis, neck tumor, Crouzon, mucopolysaccharide storage disease, hypothyroidism, Down's syndrome, excess pharyngeal collapsibility, or paradoxical glottic narrowing [1–6, 11, 12]. Other contributing factors include nasal obstruction, secretions in the airways, or airway tissue edema, as found during airway infection [13, 14].

Other causes may be superimposed on an underlying narrowing of the upper airway. *Pressure- and chemosensitive receptors* may induce apneas when saline or acid are delivered to the pharynx [15]. The mechanism may mainly concern prematures and young infants. In 3-month-old infants spontaneous acid reflux reaching the proximal portion of the thoracic esophagus was shown to be unre-

Table 2. Major causes of obstructive sleep apneas in infants

Tonsils/adenoids	14/22	Brouillette	1982
	23/32	Frank	1983
Facial dysmorphia			
Micrognathia	3/22	Brouillette	1982
Facial abnormalities	3/22	Brouillette	1982
	5/32	Frank	1983
	14/50	Guilleminault	1981
Cleft palate repair	1/22	Brouillette	1982
	2/50	Guilleminault	1981
Neurolomuscular disorders	3/32	Frank	1983
	6/50	Guilleminault	1981
General medical problems			
Hypothyroidism	1/50	Guilleminault	1981
Obesity	1/32	Frank	1983
Uncertain	1/22	Brouillette	1982
	2/50	Guilleminault	1981
'Primary' Osa syndrome	24/50	Guilleminault	1981

lated to the development of airway obstructions [16–18].

Abnormalities of the nervous system have also been associated with the development of airway obstructions. Seizure, increased intracranial pressure, and spinal cord compressions such as that associated with Chiari malformations type I or II, or syringobulbia-myelia concur to airway obstructions [1, 2, 5, 6, 19–21]. Other neurologic impairments limiting muscle contractions, such as laryngeal recurrent nerve palsy, palsy of the cranial nerves, or poliomyelitis are also associated with obstructed breathing.

The *autonomic nervous system* may play a role in apneas. Both its sympathetic and parasympathetic components could be involved [22–24]. Obstructed sleep apneas were reported in children suffering from various autonomic nervous system disorders, including familial dysautonomia, diabetes, ganglioneuroma, Shy-Drager syndrome, and breath-holding spells [25–28]. The administration of atropine has occasionally been reported to prevent obstructive sleep apneas [29, 30].

Environmental factors contribute to the development of obstructive apneas. These factors include body position, neck flexion, sleep deprivation, or the use of sedatives [31–33]. Nasal obstructions are associated with the prone position. Sedative drugs, such as those containing phenothiazines, induce obstructive apneas in infants.

Increased Airway Resistances

In adults and children, increases in airway pressures have been described, without overt obstruction. It is believed that such finding could indicate the presence of partial obstructions, and possibly, a tendency towards the development of obstructive sleep apneas [2, 21]. Such mechanisms could be at work in sleeping infants as well.

Clinical Experience with Sleep Apneas in Infants

From the literature, the major causes of obstructive sleep apneas in infants are as shown in table 2.

Table 3. Ostructive sleep apneas in otherwise healthy children

	n	%
Tonsils/adenoids	6/40	15
Laryngomalacia	6/40	15
Facial dysmorphia: choanal atresia	1/40	2.5
Nasal congestion	1/40	2.5
General medical problems		
Allergies to cow's milk	8/40	20
Allergies to soya	1/40	2.5
Allergies to dust	1/40	2.5
'Primary' Osa syndrome	16/40	40

From our own clinical experience, obstructive sleep apneas in otherwise healthy infants may be divided as shown in table 3.

Allergic reactions to cow's milk, soya, or dust may contribute to the development of hypersecretions in the airways, nasal congestion, and obstructive sleep apneas. Within 4–6 weeks of a dietary treatment with a hypoallergenic diet, the obstructive sleep apneas may disappear.

The 'primary' obstructive sleep apneas are those for whom no cause for obstructed breathing may be found.

Clinical Consequences of Obstructive Apneas

Inefficient breathing efforts induce drops in heart rates, cardiac output, and transcutaneous oxygen saturation values [23, 27, 34]. Occasional reports in children indicate that repeated obstructive apneas may lead to pulmonary edema, hypertension, and congestive heart failure. Pulmonary or systemic hypertension, and polycythemia may also develop [2, 21, 26]. Repeated obstructive apneas have also been associated with the occurrence of sudden deaths in infants [9, 35–37].

Conclusions

Obstructive sleep apneas may be due to a variety of causes. A complete and multidisciplinary work-up is needed to evaluate these infants.

Acknowledgments

We would like to thank Prof. H.L. Vis for his constant encouragement. This study was supported by the Fondation Nationale de la Recherche Scientifique (Grant 9.4524.87).

References

1 Brouillette R, Hanson D, David R, Klemka L, Szatkowski A, Fernbach S, Hunt C: A diagnostic approach to suspected obstructive sleep apnea in children. J Pediatr 1984;105:10–14.
2 Guilleminault C: Obstructive sleep apnea syndrome in children; in Guilleminault C (ed): Sleep and Its Disorders in Children. New York, Raven Press, 1987, pp 213–224.
3 Felman AH, Loughlin GM, Leftridge CA, et al: Upper airway obstruction during sleep in children. AJR 1979;133:213–216.
4 Surrat PM, Dee P, Atkinson RL, et al: Fluoroscopic and computed tomographic features of the pharyngeal airway in obstructive sleep apnea. Am Rev Resp Dis 1983;127:487–492.
5 Brouillette RT, Fernbach SK, Hunt CE: Obstructive sleep apnea in infants and children. J Pediatr 1982;100:31–40.
6 Guilleminault C, Korobkin R, et al: A review of 50 children with obstructive sleep apnea syndrome. Lung 1981;59:275–287.
7 Flores-Guevara R, Plouin P, Curzi-Dascalova L, et al: Sleep apneas in normal neonates and infants during the first 3 months of life. Neuropediatrics 1982;13:21–28.
8 Kahn A, Rebuffat E, et al: Brief airway obstructions during sleep in infants with breath-holding spells. J Pediatr 1990;117:188–193.
9 Albani M, Bentel KHP, Budde C, et al: Infant sleep apnea profile: Preterm vs. term infants. Eur J Pediatr 1985;143:261–268.

10 Kahn A, Mozin MJ, Rebuffat E, et al: Sleep pattern alterations and brief airway obstructions in overweight infants. Sleep 1989;12:430–438.
11 Guilleminault C, Helat G, Powell N, et al: Small airway in near-miss sudden infant death syndrome infants and their families. Lancet 1987;i: 402–407.
12 Southall DP, Stebbens VA, et al: Upper airway obstruction with hypoxemia and sleep disruption in Down syndrome. Dev Med Child Neurol 1987;29:734–742.
13 Abreu E Silva FA, Macfayden UM, et al: Sleep apnoea during upper respiratory infection and metabolic alkalosis in infancy. Arch Dis Child 1986;61:1056–1062.
14 Tonkin SL, Partrigde J, Beach D, et al: The pharyngeal effect of partial nasal obstruction. Pediatrics 1974; 63:261–271.
15 Pickens DL, Schefft G, Thach BT: Pharyngeal fluid clearance and aspiration preventive mechanisms in sleeping infants. J Appl Physiol 1989;66:1164–1171.
16 Kahn A, Rebuffat E, Sottiaux M, et al: Lack of temporal relation between acid reflux in the proximal oesophagus and cardiorespiratory events in sleeping infants. Eur J Pediatr 1992;151:208–212.
17 Walsh JK, Farrell MK, Keenan WJ, et al: Gastroesophageal reflux in infants: relation to apnea. J Pediatr 1981;99:197–201.
18 Ariagno RL, Guilleminault C, Baldwin R, et al: Movement and gastroesophageal reflux in awake term infants with 'near miss' SIDS, unrelated to apnea. J Pediatr 1982;100: 894–897.
19 Haponik EF, Givens D, Angelo J: Syringobulbia-myelia with obstructive sleep apnea. Neurology 1983; 33:1064–1069.
20 Kelly DH, Shannon DC: Episodic complete airway obstruction in infants. Pediatrics 1981;67:823–827.
21 Guilleminault C: Obstructive sleep apnea syndrome and its treatment in children: Areas of agreement and controversy. Pediatr Pulmonol 1987;3:429–436.
22 Sullivan CE, Grunstein RR, Marrone O, et al: Sleep apnea pathophysiology: Upper airway and control of breathing; in Guilleminault C, Partinnen M (eds): Obstructive Sleep Apnea Syndrome: Clinical Research and Treatment. New York, Raven Press, 1990, pp 49–69.
23 Thach BT, Davies AM, Koenig JS: Pathophysiology of sudden upper airway obstruction in sleeping infants and its relevance to SIDS; in Schwartz PJ, Southall DP, Valdes-Dapena M (ed): The Sudden Infant Death Syndrome. Cardiac and Respiratory Mechanisms and Interventions. New York, Annals of New York Academy of Sciences, 1988, vol 533, p 314–328.
24 Schwartz PJ: Cardiac sympathetic innervation and the sudden infant death syndrome: A possible pathological link. Am J Med 1976;60: 167–172.
25 Chokroverty S, Sachdeo R, et al: Autonomic dysfunction and sleep apnea in olivopontocerebellar degeneration. Arch Neurol 1984;41:926–931.
26 Frank Y, Kravath RE, Pollak CP: Obstructive sleep apnea and its therapy: Clinical and polysomnographic manifestations. Pediatrics 1983;71: 737–742.
27 Guilleminault C, Tilkian A, Lehrman K, et al: Sleep apnea syndrome: States of sleep and autonomic dysfunction. J Neurol Neurosurg Psychiatry 1977;40:718–724.
28 Lehrman KL, Guilleminault C, et al: Sleep apnea syndrome in a patient with Shy-Drager syndrome. Arch Intern Med 1978;138:206–209.
29 Kelly DH, Shannon DC: Episodic complete airway obstruction in infants. Pediatrics 1981;67:823–827.
30 Kahn A, Rebuffat E, Sottiaux M, et al: Prevention of airway obstructions during sleep in infants with breath-holding spells by means of oral belladonna. A prospective double-blind crossover evaluation. Sleep 1991;14:432–438.
31 Tonkin S: Airway occlusion as a possible cause of SIDS; in Robinson RR (ed): SIDS. Canadian Foundation for the Study of Infant Deaths, 1974, pp 73–75.
32 Canet E, Gaultier C, D'Allest AM, et al: Effects of sleep deprivation on respiratory events during sleep in healthy infants. J Appl Physiol 1989;66:1158–1163.
33 Kahn A, Hasaerts D, Blum D, et al: Phenothiazine-induced sleep apneas in normal infants. Pediatrics 1985; 75:844–847.
34 Kahn A, Blum D, Waterschoot P, et al: Effect of obstructive sleep apneas on transcutaneous oxygen pressure in control infants, siblings of sudden infant death syndrome victims, and near miss infants: Comparison with the effects of central sleep apneas. Pediatrics 1982;70:852–857.
35 Guilleminault C, Ariagno RL, Forno LS, et al: Obstructive sleep apneas and near miss SIDS: I. Report of an infant with sudden death. Pediatrics 1979;63:837–843.
36 Kahn A, Blum D, Rebuffat E, et al: Polysomnographic studies in infants who subsequently died of sudden infant death syndrome. Pediatrics 1988;82:721–727.
37 Kahn A, Groswasser J, Rebuffat E, et al: Sleep and cardiorespiratory characteristics of infant victims of sudden death: A prospective case-control study. Sleep 1992;15:287–292.

Biol Neonate 1994;65:240–246

J. Ramet

Pediatric and Neonatal Intensive Care Units, A.Z.-Vrije Universiteit, Brussels, Belgium

Cardiac and Respiratory Reactivity to Gastroesophageal Reflux: Experimental Data in Infants

Key Words

Gastroesophageal reflux
Cardiac reactivity
Respiratory reactivity
Acid infusion
Esophagus
Vagus nerve
Bradycardia
Apnea
Arousal

Abstract

Gastroesophageal reflux associated with apnea and/or bradycardia induces both dilatation of the esophagus and abrupt intrusion of acid content in it. To evaluate the relative importance of these two types of stimulation on cardiac and respiratory responses, a series of experimental protocols were designed, in which we evaluated the influence of esophageal dilatation alone, acid infusion alone and both stimulations simultaneously. The passage of a volume in the lower third of the esophagus (n = 14) during reflux was simulated by balloon dilatation; the passage of acid gastric juice during reflux was simulated by an esophageal acid infusion test, within the physiological range (n = 8; duration = 5 min; pH = 2.2). Cardiac, respiratory and arousal responses were compared during a control period and during the distal balloon dilatation and esophageal saline and acid infusion periods. Distal esophageal balloon dilatation and acid infusion induced significant prolongation of the RR interval and of the duration of the respiratory cycle. The presence of the esophageal catheter did not lead to continuous vagal stimulation. Simultaneous stimulation by balloon dilatation and acid infusion provoked cardiac responses that were above the level reached by each stimulation separately. Behavioral and electroencephalographic observations demonstrate significantly more frequent and longer arousal responses during the acid infusion than during control and saline infusion periods. We conclude that distal esophageal balloon dilatation and acid infusion elicit significant cardiac and respiratory responses in newborns during active sleep. Since arousal from sleep has been shown to facilitate esophageal clearance, we speculate that arousal responses, observed only during acid infusion, may be one of the defence mechanisms related to acid gastroesophageal reflux.

Introduction

Gastroesophageal reflux associated with apnea and/or bradycardia has been reported in infants [1, 2]. During gastroesophageal reflux both dilatation and the abrupt intrusion of acid content into the esophagus are observed: two phenomena are thus evoked during an acid gastroesophageal reflux. To evaluate the relative importance of these two types

Dr. J. Ramet
Pediatric and Neonatal Intensive Care Units
A.Z.-Vrije Universiteit
B–1090 Brussels (Belgium)

0006–3126/94/
0654–0240$5.00/0

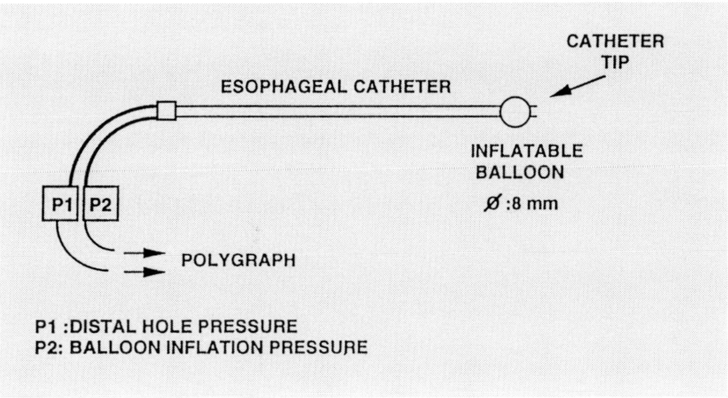

Fig. 1. Double lumen esophageal catheter with inflatable balloon.

of stimulations on the cardiac and respiratory responses, a series of experimental protocols were designed in which we, respectively, evaluated the effect of esophageal dilatation alone, of acid infusion alone and of both together.

The Esophageal Dilatation Test

Subjects and Methods

An esophageal dilatation test (EDT) was performed on 41 infants (postconceptional age 31.5–50 weeks), using a standardized technique and timing [3]. A double lumen 60-cm catheter derived from a Swan-Ganz catheter with an inflatable balloon was inserted in the lower third of the esophagus (fig. 1).

The proximal ends of the catheter were connected to two pressure transducers: P_1 or pressure at the distal hole and P_2 or the balloon inflation pressure. Several variables were polygraphically monitored: electro-encephalogram (EEG), ECG by bipolar chest leads and breathing pattern (thoracic and abdominal movements by strain gauges and nasal airflow by thermistors) (fig. 2).

Recording Schedule

Each infant was monitored during unmedicated sleep in his crib in the early morning. States of alertness were determined upon EEG and behavioral criteria. The EDT was performed during a well-established 'active' REM sleep period. The balloon was abruptly inflated and the intraballoon pressure was kept constant for 10 s prior to quick deflation.

Analysis of Cardiac Data

(1) 'Control RR' intervals: definition of terms – mean RR intervals determined from measurement of each RR interval recorded for 60 s during 'active' REM sleep just prior to and after the placement of the esophageal balloon; (2) EDT-related variables, the longest RR interval in milliseconds noted during the balloon inflation; (3) the 'percent RR (%RR)' or the longest RR interval in ms divided by mean control RR in ms multiplied by 100.

Analysis of Respiratory Data

Definition of terms: (1) 'control T_{TOT}'; (2) EDT variables: the longest T_{TOT} in seconds noted during the balloon inflation. The longest t_{TOT} included either a respiratory cycle with prolonged expiratory time or a respiratory cycle followed by a missed breath. A missed breath was defined as an absence of air-exchange for a duration equal to control T_{TOT} + 1 SD; (3) 'percent T_{TOT}' (%T_{TOT}) was calculated and involved the longest T_{TOT} during EDT divided by mean control T_{TOT} in seconds multiplied by 100.

Statistical Analysis

Paired t test was performed between the 2 control periods. Analyses between GA, PCA and measured variables were performed using linear and multiplicative regression.

Results

The two 'control variables', before and after placement of the catheter, were not statistically different, i.e. the insertion of the esoph-

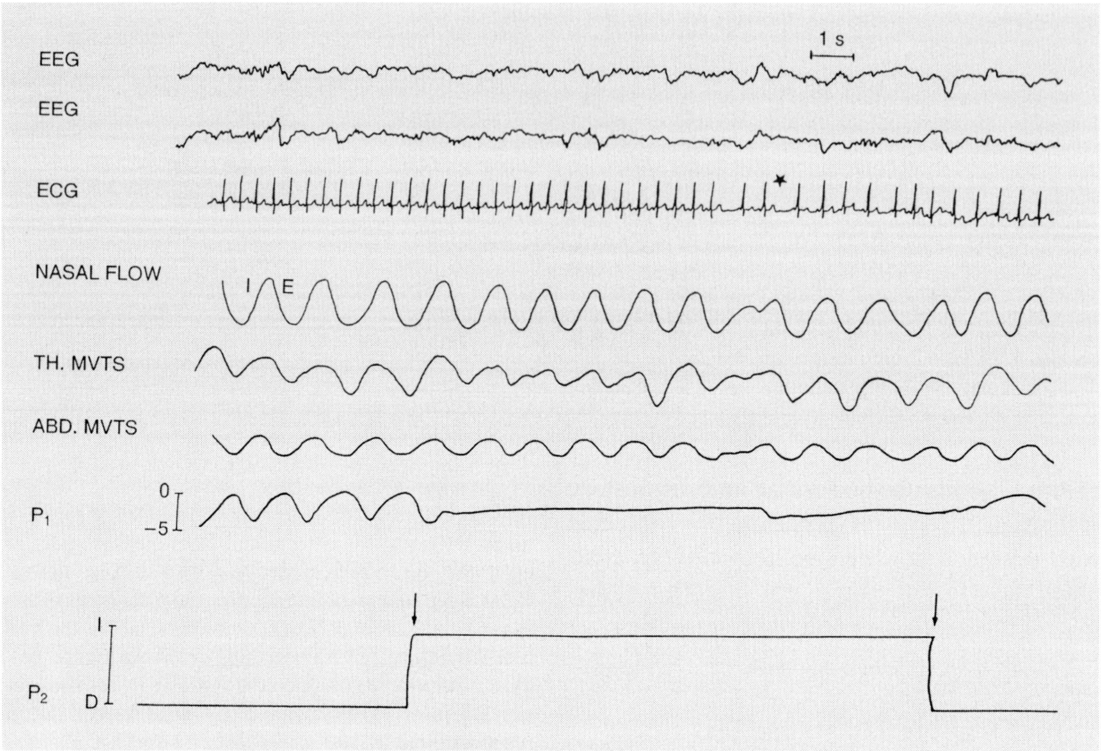

Fig. 2. Esophageal dilatation test (EDT). Top to bottom: channel 1 = EEG FP_2-C_4; channel 2 = EEG C_4-T_4; channel 3 = ECG (bipolar chest leads); channel 4 = nasal flow (I = inspiration, E = expiration); channels 5 and 6 = thoracic and abdominal movements; channel 7 = esophageal pressure (P1); channel 8 = balloon inflation pressure (P2). On the ECG tracing, the asterisk indicates the longest RR interval. On the P2 line, the arrows indicate begin and end of balloon inflation (10 s). D = Deflation; I = inflation. Loss of the P1 signal during EDT is due to the technique of pressure measurement using a Swan-Ganz catheter.

ageal apparatus in the lower esophagus did not lead to a continuous vagal stimulation. EDT provoked a prolongation of the RR interval in all infants. The cardiac responses during EDT, expressed as longest RR interval in msec, ranged from 410 to 835 ms (mean ± SD: 529.4 ± 110.5 ms). When longest RR interval during EDT was normalized, i.e. when we considered %RR, there was a statistically significant decrease of the heart rate response to the esophageal dilatation with GA ($p < 0.003$). EDT provoked a prolongation of T_{TOT} in 35 infants. When we considered $\%T_{TOT}$, there was a significant decrease with increasing PCA ($\%T_{TOT} = 2 \cdot 10^4\ PCA^{-1.33}$; $r = 0.46$; $p < 0.003$).

Discussion

Our results show that esophageal dilatation performed during 'active' REM sleep causes a prolongation of RR interval and T_{TOT} in healthy infants. The cardiac and respiratory

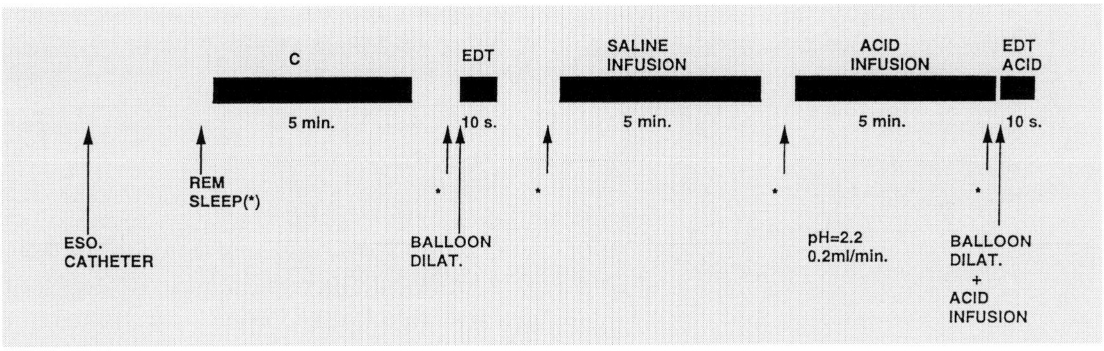

Fig. 3. The esophageal acid infusion test. Recording schedule: C = control period; EDT = esophageal dilatation test; periods of saline and acid infusion; EDT ACID = esophageal dilatation during acid infusion.

responses when normalized (for the mean control values preceding the test) decreased with advancing age. The strength of both cardiac and respiratory responses to the EDT challenge is significantly blunted with maturation.

Standardization of the method included: specific location of the stimulation at the lower third of the esophagus, precise determination of inflation pressure, onset and arrest of the test, control on maintenance of plateau level during ten seconds. Only EDT's performed during active sleep were retained, avoiding possible variations of the responses due to external factors.

The evidence for the vagal origin of this reflex is founded on its known anatomical pathways and by the fact that this reflex is abolished by anticholinergic drugs. The literature is full of anecdotal reports of neurological or cardiac symptoms secondary to esophageal disorders (organic or functional). In children, reports of 'esophageal-induced' bradyarrhythmias are less numerous. Experimental evidence obtained in adult dogs demonstrated inhibition of diaphragmatic activity, during esophageal dilatation, which could be abolished by vagotomy [5]. It could be concluded that stretch of the esophagus may be a component of induced vagally mediated reflex apnea.

The Esophageal Acid Infusion Test

Subjects and Methods

Eight healthy infants, with a postconceptional age of 36–40 weeks participated in this study. Informed parental consent was obtained and the study was approved by the institutional ethics committee. According to previously described parameters, none of these infants presented pathological gastroesophageal reflux [6].

Acid Stimulation Test

Prior to the Acid Stimulation Test all infants underwent 24-hour esophageal pH monitoring. The Acid Stimulation Test was performed during spontaneous unmedicated sleep. The test was performed using a standardized technique and timing. A catheter with an external diameter of 1.5 mm was inserted in the lower third of the esophagus. The esophageal pressure was monitored on an Alvar polygraph simultaneously with the variables described in the esophageal dilatation study.

Recording Schedule (fig. 3)

Three consecutive periods of precisely 5 min were studied: a control period followed by periods of saline and acid infusion. At the end of the acid infusion, an

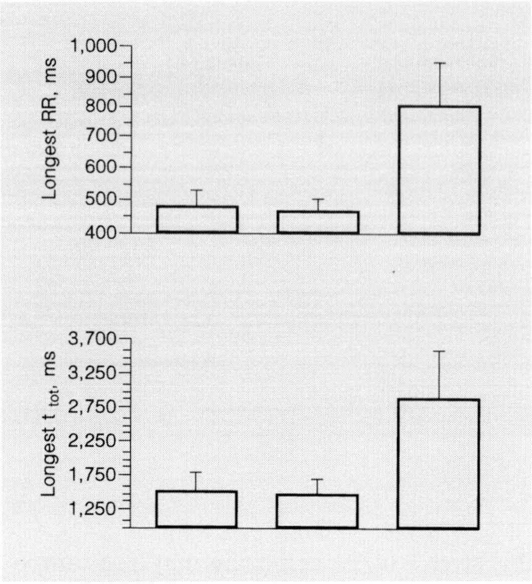

Fig. 4. Esophageal infusion test. Longest RR (upper panel) and longest T_{TOT} (lower panel) observed during control, saline and acid infusion periods; there was a significant increase in both longest RR and longest T_{TOT} during acid infusion periods when compared to control and saline infusion periods (*$p < 0.01$).

esophageal dilatation test was performed during 10 s to evaluate the effect of the simultaneous occurrence of both procedures. The level of acidity (pH = 2.2) and the duration (5 min) of the acid infusion were based on the values observed during spontaneous GER in healthy infants.

Data Analysis

Cardiac, respiratory and arousal responses were analyzed during the three consecutive periods, according to the techniques described in the first study.

Arousal Responses

Polygraphic analysis and behavioral scoring were performed to observe the occurrence of any changes in the state of alertness and specially arousal responses. Arousal from REM sleep was defined as the presence of clear flattening and desynchronization of the EEG, i.e. EEG arousal [7]. The total number of arousals (n) and the cumulative duration of arousals (s) were calculated for each period of 5 min.

A one-way analysis of variance (Anova) was performed to compare the various parameters during the three periods.

Results

Control, Saline and Acid Infusion Periods

A significant increase in mean RR and longest RR was observed when both control and saline infusion periods were compared to the acid infusion period ($p < 0.01$, fig. 4).

Respiratory Responses. The longest T_{TOT} increased significantly ($p < 0.01$) during acid infusion when compared to control and saline infusions (fig. 4).

Arousal Responses. No clinical arousal responses (opening of the eyes and awakening) was observed. Only EEG arousals occurred. Both arousal number (n) and total EEG arousal duration (s), almost nil during the control and saline infusion periods, increased significantly during the acid infusion period ($p < 0.01$).

Simultaneous Stimulation. Esophageal dilatation during acid infusion provoked a prolongation of the RR interval above the level reached during control period, during esophageal dilatation alone and during acid infusion alone. Longest T_{TOT} during dilatation and during acid infusion separately were longer than the control values, but dilatation during acid infusion did not provoke an increase above the level reached by acid infusion alone.

Discussion

This study demonstrates that, in healthy infants during REM sleep, distal esophageal acid infusion induces significant cardiac and respiratory responses and elicits significant EEG arousal responses, when compared to control or esophageal saline infusion periods. Moreover, we were able to demonstrate that esophageal dilatation during acid infusion causes a cardiac response superior to the level produced by each stimulation separately [8].

Esophageal acid infusion has been used in a wide variety of diagnostic situations in infants and adults [9, 10]. In these studies, prolonged acid infusions or very low pH were used. In the present study, for evident ethical reasons, the level of acidity and the duration of the acid infusion were precisely controlled at a level selected to match the mean duration of the longest reflux observed in healthy infants. Thus the acid esophageal stimulation was within physiological range. Our data show that preterm infants in REM sleep have EEG arousal responses to distal mild acid infusion.

Since arousal from sleep has been shown to facilitate acid esophageal clearance, arousal is presumably a mechanism that protects from severe cardiac and/or respiratory events. Thus, it may be speculated that, in infants with bradycardia and/or apnea, GER-related severe cardiac and respiratory events are due to a deficient arousal response to acid esophageal stimulation and delayed acid clearance. Deficiency in arousal response to acid stimulation during sleep may have several underlying mechanisms. Moreover, it has been demonstrated that circadian rhythms also influence the responses to vagal stimulation tests [11].

Nonhuman and human studies have shown that sleep deprivation and sleep fragmentation modifies the threshold of arousal responses to respiratory stimuli [12]. Clinical experience indicated that infants and children with GER had disturbances in sleep and awakening, and duration of sleep increases with treatment of the reflux [13]. Moreover, arousal deficiency has been observed in some near-miss SIDS infants [14].

General Conclusion

We evaluated by a series of investigational procedures the cardiac and respiratory responses to acid gastroesophageal reflux. Both esophageal dilatation and esophageal acid infusion were performed separately and simultaneously to simulate the two components of acid gastroesophageal reflux. The cardiac and respiratory responses during balloon dilatation and during acid infusion were respectively more important than during control and saline infusion periods. The presence of the esophageal catheter did not lead to a continuous vagal stimulation. When compared to other vagal stimulation tests, the cardiac responses to the esophageal dilatation alone may be considered as mild [15, 16]. Significant prolongation of the RR and T_{TOT} intervals were observed during acid infusion. Simultaneous stimulation by balloon dilatation and acid infusion provoked cardiac responses that were above the level reached by each stimulation separately. Quite unexpectedly, behavioral and electroencephalographical observation permitted to demonstrate arousal responses that were significantly more frequent and longer than during control and saline infusion periods. Since arousal from sleep has been shown to facilitate esophageal clearance, we may speculate that the arousal responses, observed in our investigation, may be one of the defense mechanisms related to acid gastroesophageal reflux.

References

1 Herbst JJ, Book LS, Bray PF: Gastroesophageal reflux in the near miss sudden infant death syndrome. J Pediatr 1978;92:73–75.

2 Herbst JJ, Minton SD, Book LS: Gastroesophageal reflux causing respiratory distress and apnea in newborn infants. J Pediatr 1979;95: 763–768.

3 Ramet J, Praud JP, d'Allest AM, Dehan M, Guilleminault C, Gaultier Cl: Cardiac and respiratory responses to esophageal dilatation during REM sleep in human infants. Biol Neonate 1988;58:181–187.

4 Schey WL, Meus P, Levinsky RA, Campbell C, Replogle R: Esophageal dysmotility and the sudden infant death syndrome. Experimental observations of neonatal puppies. Radiology 1981;140:73–77.

5 Cherniack NS, Haxtriu MA, Mitra J, Strohl K, Van Lunteren E: Responses of upper airway, intercostal and diaphragm muscle activity to stimulation of esophageal afferent in dogs. J Physiol 1984;349:15–25.

6 Dreizzen E, Escourrou P, Odievre M, Guilleminault C, Gaultier Cl: Esophageal reflux in symptomatic and asymptomatic infants: Postprandial and circadian variations. J Pediatr Gastroenterol Nutr 1990; 10:316–321.

7 Monod N, Garma L: Auditory responsivity in the human premature. Biol Neonate 1971;17:292–316.

8 Ramet J, Egreteau L, Curzi-Dascalova L, Dehan M, Gaultier Cl: Cardiac, respiratory, and arousal responses to an esophageal acid infusion test in near-term infants during active sleep. J Pediatr Gastroenterol Nutr 1992;15:135–140.

9 Berezin S, Medow MS, Glassman M, Newman LJ: Use of the intraesophageal acid perfusion test in provoking non-specific chest pain in children. J Pediatr 1989;115:709–712.

10 Helm JF, Dodds WJ, Pelc LR, Palmer DW, Hogan WJ, Teeter BD: Effect of esophageal emptying and saliva on clearance of acid from the esophagus. N Engl J Med 1984;310: 284–288.

11 Ramet J, Hauser B, Waldura J, De Prins J: Circadian rhythm of cardiac responses to vagal stimulation tests. Pediatr Neurol 1992;8:91–96.

12 Guilleminault C, Rosekind M: The arousal threshold: sleep deprivation, sleep fragmentation, and obstructive sleep apnea syndrome. Bull Eur Physiopathol Respir 1981;17:341–349.

13 Shepherd RW, Wren J, Evans S, Lander M, Ong TH: Gastroesophageal reflux in children, clinical profile, course and outcome with active therapy in 126 cases. Clin Pediatr 1987;26:55–60.

14 Van Der Hal AL, Rodriguez AM, Sargent CW, Platzker ACG, Keens TG: Hypoxic and hypercapnic arousal responses and prediction of subsequent apnea in apnea of infancy. Pediatrics 1985;75:848–854.

15 Ramet J, Praud JP, d'Allest AM, et al: Effect of maturation on heart rate response to ocular compression test during rapid eye movement sleep in human infants. Pediatr Res 1988; 24:477–480.

16 Ramet J, Praud JP, d'Allest AM, Dehan M, Gaultier Cl: Trigeminal airstream stimulation. Maturation-related cardiac and respiratory responses during REM sleep in human infants. Chest 1990;98:92–96.

Biol Neonate 1994;65:247–251

Pierre Monin

Inserm Unité, 272, Université Nancy 1, Faculté de Médecine, Nancy, France

Modifications of Ventilatory Reflexes: An Efficient Therapy for Apneas of Prematurity?

Key Words

Ventilatory reflexes
Apneas
Prematurity
Continuous positive airways pressure

Abstract

The treatment of apneas of prematurity mainly involves the use of drugs (methylxanthines, doxapram). Despite evidence of the efficacy, some adverse effects may occur raising the question of other therapies. This brief review analyses the usefulness of methods influencing the ventilatory reflexes: cutaneous and proprioceptive stimulation and nasal continuous positive airways pressure proposed previously.

Immaturity of the respiratory system is associated with a high risk for apnea in the premature infant. The reason is multifactorial and partly supported by a decrease in central respiratory drive, in the activity of ventilatory reflexes and by the generation of apnea reflexes in response to modifications of the ventilatory system (chest distorsion, decrease in lung volume). Despite the great efficacy of the pharmacological treatment for apneas with methylxanthines or doxapram, some methods influencing the ventilatory reflexes have also been proposed in the treatment of apneic premature babies [1–3]. The aim of this short review is to analyze if such methods should still be used and recommended.

The Ventilatory Reflexes

The respiratory control is modulated by humoral and neurogenic afferents of either central and intercentral or reflex origin.

Reflexes of Pulmonary Origin

Three type of receptors are involved in these reflexes. The strech receptors located in the airways muscles and stimulated by lung distension are responsible for the so-called Hering-Breuer reflex inhibiting the inspiration with the increase in lung volume. This reflex is present in the term neonate [4] and is greater in the premature baby [5, 6]. It has been shown to be attenuated in apneic premature babies [7]. Irritant receptors located in

Pierre Monin
Inserm Unité 272
Université Nancy 1
Faculté de Médecine
F–54013 Nancy (France)

0006–3126/94/
0654–0247$5.00/0

the epithelial cells from the trachea to the alveolar ducts are stimulated by irritating substances, the contractions of the airways and the changes in lung volume. An overdistension induces the head paradoxical reflex observed in the neonate [4]; a deflation of the lung induces the Hering-Breuer deflation reflex. These reflexes induce an increase in inspiratory activity and are immature in the premature infant [8]. A paradoxical response with an increase in inspiratory activity followed by an apnea can be observed. The juxtacapillary receptors (J receptors) are also stimulated by irritating substances, edema and pulmonary congestion. These receptors are developed postnatally; their stimulation induces also an increase in ventilation.

Extrapulmonary Reflexes

Ventilation is also influenced by reflexes of extrapulmonary origin. Spinal proprioceptive reflexes are generated by the stimulation of thoracic mechanoreceptors of the neuromuscular spindles of intercostal muscles and to a lesser extent of the diaphragm. These proprioceptive afferents may alter the phrenic nerve activity [9].

They can be generated by the distorsion of the rib cage particularly during REM sleep and may play a role in the pathogenesis of apneas by induction of an early arrest of inspiratory activity. Somatic proprioceptive receptors located in the somatic muscles of the limbs [10] and in joints [11] are also responsible for an increase in ventilation. A passive mobilisation of the limbs induces an increase in ventilation [12]. This reflex has been demonstrated in the neonatal period in the rabbit [13].

The stimulation of the cutaneous receptors also induces an increase in ventilation [14]. This type of stimulation may also modify the respiratory control by the induction of arousal since quiet and REM sleep have been shown to be more vulnerable states than wakefulness to the development of reflex apneas. Other afferents from nasal pharyngeal and laryngeal receptors can also modify respiratory control and induce a drop in respiratory frequency and apneas in the neonate [15–17]. The immaturity and/or the induction of these reflexes are considered as possible mechanisms for the development of apnea of prematurity. Thus, any method increasing afferents to the respiratory centers or reducing apnea-triggering reflexes can be considered as a possible therapy. Therefore, it is difficult to separate the effects of methods such as cutaneous and/or proprioceptive stimulation and nasal continuous positive airways pressure (CPAP) from the effects of other nursing procedures (posture, temperature adjustments, number of blood sampling, etc.).

Methods Influencing the Ventilatory Reflexes

Cutaneous and Proprioceptive Stimulation

The stimulation of cutaneous proprioceptive receptors has long been proposed on the basis of empirical observations. This method inducing an increase in afferents to the respiratory center has been clearly documented in apneic premature babies by Kattwinkel et al. [3] in 1975. The increase in afferents depends also on arousal induced by cutaneous stimulation. The influence of arousal on respiratory control has been studied extensively and its positive effect on the frequency of apnea is well documented [18]. Somatic proprioceptive receptors can also be stimulated by the use of oscillating waterbeds [2]. This method simulating the stimulations received by the fetus in utero has been shown initially to significantly reduce apnea frequency and also to provide better growth and development [19]. However, in a controlled study Jones [20] showed the absence of any significant effect of a similar oscillating waterbed. In 1982, Tuck et al. [21] demonstrated using only an oscillating regular bed in order to provide vestibular stimulation and a significant reduction in apnea frequency (table 1). The problem was reevaluated by Saigal et al. [22] in 1985 who, in a first study, showed a lower effect than with theophylline therapy.

Table 1. Influence of an oscillating bed on the occurrence of apnea and bradycardia in premature infants

	Total number of events recorded			Infants for whom event was more frequent	
	rocking	control	p	in rocking period	in control period
Apnea (>12 s)	69	119	<0.001	1	11
Apnea with bradycardia (<100/min)	58	101	<0.01	1	9
Apnea with fall in $TcPO_2$ to below 50 mm Hg	17	51	<0.005	1	8
Apnea requiring additional stimulation	6	28	<0.05	1	5

A significant drop is observed in all but 1 patient. Note the dramatic decrease of apneas requiring additional stimulation. From Tuck et al. [21].

Table 2. Apneic attack rates during treatment (percentage of pretreatment rates)

	Theophylline median (range)	CPAP median (range)	Significance
1st day of treatment, all attacks ≥10 s	15	43	0.05 < 0.1
(n = 18 and 14)	(0–83)	(0–698)	
Whole course of treatment, all attacks ≥10 s	14	45	p = 0.05
(n = 18 and 14)	(0–72)	(0–698)	
1st day of treatment, prolonged attacks ≥20 s	0	57	p < 0.01
(n = 10 and 10)	(0.64)	(0.408)	
Whole course of treatment, prolonged attacks ≥60 s	0	52	p < 0.05
(n = 11 and 10)	(0–>100)	(0–408)	

Comparative effect of theophylline therapy and CPAP. The difference is particularly important for severe apneas. From Jones [25].

In a second study performed on a larger number of patients, using an oscillating air mattress, there was no significant effect of this method of treatment on apnea frequency and they concluded to the limited usefulness of this method. Therefore, considering these contradictory data and the different types of stimulation (oscillating waterbed, oscillating bed, air mattress with longitudinal wave motion), it seems reasonable to re-evaluate the effects of oscillations in order to exclusively provide a vestibular stimulation as in the Tuck et al. [21] study which showed a significant effect using a crossover design. The mechanisms of action of the oscillating waterbed are not yet fully understood [23].

Continuous Positive Airways Pressure

Proposed in the mid-seventies to prevent apnea of prematurity, nasal CPAP stabilizes the rib cage and increases lung volume. Its efficacy on apneas is well documented. The stabilisation of the rib cage probably reduces apneas triggering reflexes generated by stimulation of the thoracic proprioceptive receptors. CPAP also modify the afferents to the respiratory centers. By the occlusion method, this technique has been shown to influence the activity of the inhibitory inspiratory reflex of Hering-Breuer reduced in apneic patients. The prolongation of inspiration of the first breath post-occlusion might also be the result of an elimination of

Table 3. Preventive effects of CPAP on apnea in premature infants during the weaning period [from Andreasson et al., 27]

	No CPAP (0 cm H_2O) $\overline{X} \pm SD$	CPAP (4 cm H_2O) $\overline{X} \pm SD$	Significance of difference (p value)
Transcutaneous PO_2, kPa	8.0 ± 3.0	11.1 ± 4.1	0.001
Number of apneas in 10 min	2.4 ± 3.6	0.5 ± 0.7	0.006

the Hering-Breuer deflation reflex allowing better adaptation to a respiratory load [24]. The effects of CPAP may also depend on the reduction of lung edema and on the rise in lung volume providing an increase in PaO_2 and better oxygenation of the respiratory centers. However, CPAP is less effective than theophylline therapy (table 2) [25].

This method is particularly effective on mixed and obstructive apneas as demonstrated by Miller et al. [26] and recently Andreasson et al. [27] have shown the benefit of this method in the prevention of apneas during the weaning period in babies recovering from respiratory distress (table 3).

Conclusion

From these studies, there is a lot of evidence to support the efficacy of cutaneous proprioceptive stimulation and CPAP in apnea of prematurity. The effect of a vestibular proprioceptive stimulation has not yet been confirmed and other studies utilizing a well-defined stimulation might be useful.

Considering the efficacy of the pharmacological treatment, it is not appropriate to propose these methods as alternative therapies. However, in the case of moderate apneas without significant hypoxemia they can obviously be recommended in association with appropriate nursing procedures. In clinical practice, cutaneous and proprioceptive stimulations are used empirically in premature babies developing apnea as soon as they are diagnosed by nurses. These methods might delay and, in some instances, avoid using drugs with potential adverse effects. Recently, a potentiation of airway responsiveness to caffeine, which is a frequent sequellae in premature infants, has been demonstrated in newborn lambs [28]. The real benefit of CPAP during the weaning period should also be strongly considered. Prior to the use of drugs, if adequately used these techniques can provide a real benefit as the first step in the therapeutic strategy.

References

1 Kattwinkel J: Neonatal apnea: Pathogenesis and therapy. J Pediatr 1977;90:342–347.
2 Korner A, Guilleminault C, Van den Hoed V, Baldwin R: Reduction of sleep apnea and bradycardia in preterm infants on oscillating water beds: A controlled polygraphic study. Pediatrics 1978;61:528–533.
3 Kattwinkel J, Nearman HS, Fanaroff A, Katona P, Klaus M: Apnea of prematurity: Comparative therapeutic effects of cutaneous stimulation and nasal continuous positive airway pressure. J Pediatr 1975;86: 588–592.
4 Cross KW, Klaus M, Tooley W, Weisser K: The response of the newborn baby to inflation of the lungs. J Physiol (Lond) 1960;151:551–565.
5 Bodegard G, Schwieler GH: Control of respiration in newborn babies. II. The development of the thoracic reflex response to an added respiratory load. Acta Paediatr Scand 1971; 60:181–186.
6 Bodegard G, Schwieler G, Skoglunds S, Zetterström R: Control of repiration in newborn babies. I. Development of the Hering-Breuer Inflation reflex. Acta Paediatr Scand 1969;58:567–571.

7 Gerhardt T, Bancalari E: Apnea of prematurity. II. Respiratory reflexes. Pediatrics 1984;74:63–66.
8 Flemming PJ, Bryan H: Functional immaturity of pulmonary irritant receptors and apnea in newborn preterm infants. Pediatrics 1978;31: 515–518.
9 Remmers JE, Marttila I: Action of intercostal muscle afferents on the respiratory rhythm of anesthetized cats. Respir Physiol 1975;24:31–41.
10 Bessou P, Dejours P, Laporte Y: Effets ventilatoires reflexes de la stimulation des fibres de grand diamètre, d'origine musculaire chez le chat. CR Soc Biol (Paris) 1959;153: 477–481.
11 Flandrois R, Lacour JR, Islas-Maroquin J, Charlot J: Limbs mechanoreceptors inducing the reflex hyperpnea of exercise Respir Physiol 1967;2:335–345.
12 Harrison TR, Harrison WG, Calhoun JA, Marsh JP: Congestive heart failure. XVII. The mechanism of dyspnea on exertion. Arch Intern Med 1932;50:690–720.
13 Ethevenot G: Reponse ventilatoire du lapin nouveau-né a la mobilisation passive des membres; thèse médecine, Nancy, 1973, pp 1–161.
14 Marlot D, Duron B: Stimulation cutanée et activité respiratoire spontanée chez le chaton; in Duron B (éd): Colloque INSERM: Centres respiratoires et systèmes afférents, 1976, pp 273–280.
15 Haddad G, Mellins R: The role of airways receptors in the control of respiration: A review. J Pediatr 1977;91:281–286.
16 Duron B, Marlot D: Evolution des réflexes d'Hering-Breuer au cours de la periode néo-natale chez le chaton; in Duron B (éd): Colloque INSERM: Centres respiratoires et Systèmes afférents, 1976, pp 282–286.
17 Downing SE, Lee JC: Laryngeal chemosensitivity: A possible mechanism for sudden infant death. Pediatrics 1975;55:647–649.
18 Marchal F, Corke B, Sundell H: Reflex apnea from laryngeal chemostimulation in the sleeping premature newborn lamb. Pediatr Res 1982;16:621–627.
19 Kramer L, Pierpont M: Rocking waterbeds and auditory stimuli to enhance growth of preterm infants. J Pediatr 1976;88:297–299.
20 Jones R: A controlled trial of a regularly cycled oscillating waterbed and a non-oscillating waterbed in the prevention of apnoea in the preterm infant. Arch Dis Child 1981;56: 889–891.
21 Tuck S, Monin P, Duvivier C, May T, Vert P: Effect of a rocking bed on apnoea of prematurity. Arch Dis Child 1982;57:475–477.
22 Saigal S, Watts J, Campbell D: Randomized clinical trial of an oscillating air mattress in preterm infants: Effect on apnea, growth, and development.
23 Korner A: What we don't know about water beds and apneic preterm infants. Pediatrics 1981;68: 306–307.
24 Martin R, Nearman H, Katona P, Klaus M: The effect of a low continuous positive airway pressure on the reflex control of respiration in the preterm infant. J Pediatr 1977;90: 976–981.
25 Jones R: Apnea of immaturity. 1. A controlled trial of theophylline and face mask continuous positive airways pressure. Arch Dis Child 1982; 57:761–765.
26 Miller M, Carlo W, Martin R: Continuous positive airway pressure selectively reduces obstructive apnea in preterm infants. J Pediatr 1985; 106:91–94.
27 Andreasson B, Lindroth M, Svenningsen N, Jonson B: Effects on respiration of CPAP immediately after extubation in the very preterm infant. Pediatr Pulmonol 1988;4:213–218.
28 Keklikian N, Wolfson MR, Shaffer Th: Caffeine potentiates airways responsiveness in the neonatal lamb. Pediatr Pulmonol 1992;12:17–22.

Biol Neonate 1994;65:252–257

Marie-Jeanne Boutroy

Inserm U272,
Université de Nancy I, Nancy,
France

Drug-Induced Apnea

Key Words

Apnea
Development
Drug
Neonate
Infant

Abstract

Drugs have been in the past and will in the future still be liable to induce apnea in neonates, infants and older children. At these different stages of development, the child may be abnormally vulnerable to respiratory disorders and apnea, and doses of drugs, without any abnormal side effects in adult patients, can be harmful in younger subjects. Drugs responsible for apnea during development are numerous, but more than half of the problems are induced by sedatives and hypnotics, among which phenothiazines, barbiturates, benzodiazepines (included transplacentally acquired) and general anesthetics are a few. Other pharmacological families are apnea inducers in the neonatal period and childhood: analgesics and opioid narcotics, agents acting at the levels of neuromuscular function and autonomic ganglia, and cardiovascular agents. The pathogenesis of these apneas depends on the disturbance of any mechanism responsible for the respiratory activity: medullary centers and brain stem structures, afferent influx to CNS, sleep stages, upper airways, lungs and respiratory muscles.

At key stages such as birth and infancy, drugs may emphasize the particular sensitivity of the mechanisms responsible for inducing apnea. This might explain unexpected respiratory disorders during development.

The reports of drug-induced apnea during development lead to a large chapter of the therapeutic side effects. The medical literature describes a wide variety of accidents observed in clinical trials or as anecdotal events. Apnea may occur during medical practice at home or in hospital, or still after drug antenatal exposure or acute poisoning. Three questions should be asked: (1) Which drugs are reported to have induced apnea? (2) How do they act? (3) Who is more likely to develop apnea with them?

Drugs

Sedatives and Hypnotics

This pharmacological family is responsible for more than half of apneas and respiratory disorders induced by drugs in neonates, infants or children.

Phenothiazines have been suspected to play a role in sudden infant death syndrome (SIDS), after being considered for a long time as safe for infants and commonly used for treatment of night jitteriness of nasopharyngitis. In a prospective study, Kahn et al. [1]

Marie-Jeanne Boutroy
Inserm U272
Université de Nancy I
30, rue Lionnois
F–54013 Nancy Cedex (France)

0006–3126/94/
0654–0252$5.00/0

demonstrated the role of a therapeutic dose of promethazine (1 mg/kg/day for 3 days) in affecting sleep and respiratory activity of 4 healthy infants (mean age 15.8 weeks): total sleep time increased by 12.5%, self-arousals decreased by 67.9%, NREM I decreased and NREM III increased in each infant, central apneas increased by 39.3%, and obstructive apneas, not observed in any case prior to receiving promethazine, were observed in all 4 subjects after promethazine administration. These events were accompanied by a temporary decrease in $TcPO_2$. Recently, phenothiazine-associated apnea in two siblings was reported [2].

The use of barbiturates in children as sedative-hypnotic has declined dramatically due to their lack of specificity of effect on the central nervous system. That might explain the scarcity or reported events. However, phenobarbital keeps its usefulness as an anticonvulsant, and one must keep in mind that, when intravenously infused, it may lead to laryngospasm. Nowadays, the risk of barbiturate-associated apnea should be very low in children, even during induction for anesthesia [3, 4].

Transplacentally acquired benzodiazepines had been responsible for numerous respiratory accidents in the neonatal period within the last 20 years: diazepam [5, 6], lorazepam [6], clorazepate [6, 7], oxazepam [6], bromazepam [7], clonazepam [8]. The placental transfer of these agents is wide and fast and generally maternal dosage was high and treatment duration rather long, but at that age, so sensitive for developing apnea, low plasma concentrations have been shown to be related to respiratory depression in neonates [9].

General anesthetics are well known to give apnea at induction for anesthesia or during surgical procedures when the patients are breathing freely. Chloral hydrate, ketamine and pentazocine, widely used in the 1970s, have been moved into more recently marketed agents: propofol or etomidate. All have been shown as likely to induce apnea [3, 10–14].

Analgesics and Opioid Narcotics

Nonsteroid anti-inflammatory drugs are rarely responsible for respiratory disorders in children; the risk of a severe encephalopathy with salicylates is known and exceptional, apart from heavy accidental poisoning. Ibuprofen seems safer than salicylates: Hall et al. [15] described only 7% of children (10 months to 5 years) which became symptomatic after ibuprofen overdose, suffering with central nervous depression, seizures, apnea, brachycardia, and until death in 1 case. Contrary to adults, in whom the history of amount of ibuprofen is not predictive of the potential for developing symptoms, in children, there is a statistically significant correlation between the mg/kg amount ingested and the development of symptoms (> 99 mg/kg).

Morphine and related (heroin, codeine) drugs depress respiration in adults, children and neonates, even with doses too small to disturb conciousness. The same pattern exists for meperidine or pethidine, fentanyl and alfentanil, as well as for methadone, normethadone and propoxyphene [16–19], and for opioids with mixed actions (agonist-antagonist and partial agonists) like pentazocine and nalbuphine [20]. Not only may they induce apnea, but also, the number and total duration of apnea is dose related [16]. In infants born to treated mothers, the opioids may represent an added risk to hypoxia, frequently observed in the neonatal period. Stephen et al. [21] showed, in the newborn rabbit, that the duration of primary apnea induced by acute anoxia was increased, and that death occurred more rapidly when the animals were given pethidine. The risk of agonist-antagonist opioids is growing for the neonates, because of the use of self-analgesia during labor with this last kind of mixed opioid, whose respiratory depressive effect stays at a generally safe steady state for the mothers. Unfortunately, the placental transfer of nalbuphine when given in continuous infusion, is very fast, and maternal equilibrium is reached in 15–20 min, opposite to morphine or pethidine. Moreover, this κ-agonist is badly antagonized by naloxone opposite to a μ-agonist. These pharmacological specificities seem to explain the severe respiratory depression observed in neonates born to mothers given nalbuphine.

Agents Acting at the Neuromuscular Function and Autonomic Ganglia

Neuromuscular blocking agents are used in intensive care units and for anesthesia. Their effects on respiratory movement depression and/or arrest are generally looked for according to the patients' disease. However, in some cases, respiration recovery is not obtained in the postoperative period. These problems may not always be due directly and/or only to these agents, because numerous factors are usually mixed up with those of the drugs, such as alterations in body temperature and electrolyte imbalance. Unexpected apneas induced by competitive neuromuscular blocking agents (tubocurarine, gallamine, pancuronium, fazadinium) are infrequent. The effects of fazadinium and pancuronium on respiratory functions were evaluated in children aged 6 months to 12 years [22]: the speed, depth and duration were dose related, and the duration of apnea increased significantly with increasing dosage. Much more frequent is apnea as a consequence of depolarizing agents, especially succinylcholine and suxamethonium, even in the very early ages of life [23, 24].

Some of the ganglionic neurotransmission acting agents with nicotinic specificity for cholinergic receptor sites on autonomic ganglia, are responsible for toxic respiratory failure. Tobacco products, among which are gums used for smoking abstinence (Nicorette®), may be considered as drugs and are potentially hazardous to toddlers, even if ingested in small amounts. Seizures with depressed respiration have been observed [25] after suspected oral ingestion of Nicorette or cigarette butts and verified by urine toxicology.

Apnea induced by *local anesthetics* like tetracaine, lidocaine and cocaine have seldomly been reported [26, 27]. Cocaine exposure in the antenatal period or by breast-feeding may also lead to apnea and seizures [28, 29].

Cardiovascular Drugs

Antihypertensives have been responsible for apnea in very different circumstances: accidental massive ingestion of clonidine [30, 31], anecdotal case report of administration of a collyre with timolol [32]. Neonates, as well as experimental animals and humans suffered apnea, hypoventilation and seizures during prostaglandin (A and E) infusion, often at the initial time of therapy. Hallidie-Smith [33] found a dose/respiratory effects relationship, the apnea beginning at a dose of 0.05–0.1 μg/kg/min. Finally, acute poisoning with antiarrhythmics (disopyramide) has been able to produce apnea and death.

Miscellaneous Agents

The list might be very long, but badly documented case reports and implications of other agents makes one very cautious to attribute the observed effects to a given drug. However, it seems true that iodated agents, antiparasitic drugs (chloroquine, niaprozine) and surfactant have induced apnea. For surfactant, comments must be added, because apnea should be related less to a direct pharmacologic effect than to an indirect consequence on the outcome of the group given surfactant; indeed, the survival of a large number of premature neonates freely breathing and not administered curare was more favorable to observe apneas than in the control/air group where mortality rate, mechanical ventilation and pancuronium use was higher [34].

Pathogenesis and Mechanisms

These very numerous drugs call for different components of respiratory activity for inducing apnea and, very often, several mechanisms can be intricated for the same drug.

Medullary Centers

When the drugs induce apneas by affecting medullary centers and brain stem structures, it will be generally by the way of a general depression. Several mechanisms may thus be implicated: (a) Enhancement of inhibition and decrease of facilitation mechanisms throughout the CNS, at synapsis where neurotransmission is mediated by GABA (barbiturates). (b) Increase of binding to inhibition receptors such as ω- and μ_2-receptors (benzodiazepines and morphine-like). (c) Interferences with catecholamine activity: antagonism of dopamine-mediated synaptic neurotransmision and affinity for D_2-receptors (phenothiazines), recapture blockade of norepinephrine at the terminal nerve end and in the locus ceruleus, putative center of arousal responsiveness (cocaine), agonist α_2-adrenoceptor activity on inhibitory CNS neurons (clonidine). (d) Increase in the binding percentage of benzodiazepines and GABA (barbiturates). (e) Potentiation of the sedative and respiratory depressant effect of opioids (phenothiazines, clonidine).

Excitement may still occur instead of sedation by: (a) depression of inhibitory centers (barbiturates); (b) inhibition of GABA release (morphine), and (c) excitation of central nicotine receptors (nicotine).

In those cases, and for a high extent of stimulation, seizures and apnea will be observed.

Afferent Influx

Afferent influx to CNS centers are always lessened by drugs inducing apneas: (a) respiratory and chemoreceptor drive (barbiturates); (b) hypoxic drive (barbiturates, benzodiazepines, hypnotics, opioids, iodine); (c) responsiveness to CO_2 (morphine, iodine, β-blockers); (d) arousal response (phenothiazines, cocaine).

Sleep Stages

Drug-induced central or obstructive apnea occur during sleep: (a) by increasing CNS sedation and consequently respiratory drive disturbances formerly observed during drug-free sleep, or (b) by affecting the sleep stages, especially REM sleep, during which hypotonia is very important.

After drug administration, one observes: (1) an increase in total sleep duration (barbiturates, phenothiazines, benzodiazepines); (2) a decrease or an increase in REM sleep time (barbiturates, according to whether they are given acutely or chronically), and (3) a decrease in spontaneous arousal (phenothiazine, imidazopyridines).

Upper Airways, Lungs and Respiratory Muscles

Respiratory disorders associated with drug administration may also be subsequent to constriction or relaxation: (a) upper airway muscle relaxation (phenothiazines, barbiturates, benzodiazepines, imidazopyridines, chloral hydrate); (b) laryngospasm (barbiturates, morphine); (c) increase in airways resistance by β_2-adrenoceptor blockade (β-blockers) or by histamine release (curares); (d) chest wall rigidity (opioids); (e) respiratory neuromuscular blockade (curare, suxamethonium, nicotine, anticholinesterases, local anesthetics, benzodiazepines).

Specific Aspects during Development

These drugs, responsible for apnea by the way of multiple mechanisms, act at ages and in patients more liable to develop respiratory side effects than adults.

Key Ages for Respiratory Disorders and Apnea

The neonatal period is a high-risk period for ventilatory control problems because structures and mechanisms are immature: afferent influx, so important for respiratory rhythm, lungs and upper airways, sleep stages. These peculiarities lead to specific aspects in ventilatory control, more favorable for developing central or obstructive apneas: (a) high percentage of paradoxical sleep; (b) decrease $TcPO_2$ during paradoxical sleep (until 7 months of post-natal age); (c) biphasic response to hypoxia; (d) obstructive apneas (increasing until 6 weeks of life).

These risks will be added to the specific disorders of prematurity: (a) depressed ventilatory response to hypoxia and hypercapnia; (b) vagal pulmonary tract afferences, inducing apnea (before 35 weeks' gestational age).

High-Risk Patients and Circumstances

Some patients are still at risk of respiratory impairments later than the early neonatal period. For instance, the near-miss SIDS exhibit depressed hypoxic ventilatory and bad arousal responses; the bronchodysplasic infants have a rather good arousal response, which is followed by a sustained apnea. In some congenital birth defects such as meningomyeloceles, there is a marked change in carbon dioxide and oxygen ventilatory response curves. In such cases, doses of sedatives within the therapeutic range may induce apnea. As observed in upper respiratory tract infection, obstructive apneas are much more frequent during snoring sleep than in silent sleep; they are accompanied by falls in arterial oxygen saturation (SaO_2), and its seems life-threatening to give the snoring infants drugs likely to worsen their respiratory troubles. Finally, one must keep in mind that the mode of therapy itself may lead to unexpected effects: for example, during chronic administration, therapeutic effects might change from sedation to excitation, but also drug association might enhance the probability to observe apnea: benzodiazepines administered in combination with opioids.

Drug Sensitivity in Pediatric Patients

Rarely, pediatric patients exhibit less sensitivity to drugs than adults; i.e. some general anesthetics as, for instance, propofol, for which dose requirements to obtain apnea are larger in subjects <2 years old than in older. Conversely, as with clonidine, competitive neuromuscular blocking agents, opioids and cocaine, there seems to be evidence that neonates are generally more sensitive to certain drugs, since exposure to usual or even to very low amounts are responsible for apnea. In such cases, possible pharmacokinetic mechanisms might be involved in this increased sensitivity.

To conclude, it is unquestionable that drugs have been in the past and will in the future still be liable to induce apnea in neonates, infants and older children. All the mechanisms involved in respiratory activity may be impaired by these drugs. They are given to patients going through developmental changes and who are abnormally vulnerable to respiratory disorders and apnea. Doses which are harmless in adult subjects could be harmful in younger ones.

References

1 Kahn A, Hasaerts D, Blum D: Phenothiazine-induced sleep apneas in normal infants. Pediatrics 1985;75: 844–847.
2 Buck ML, Blumer JL: Phenothiazine associated apnea in two siblings. DICP 1991;25:244–246.
3 Purcell-Jones G, Yates A, Baker JR, et al: Comparison of the induction characteristics of thiopentone and propofol in children. Br J Anaesth 1987;59:1431–1436.
4 Laishley RS, O'Callaghan AC, Lerman J: Effects of dose and concentration of rectal methohexitone for induction of anaesthesia in children. Can Anaesth Soc J 1986;33:427–432.
5 André M, Sibout M, Pétry JM, et al: Dépression respiratoire et neurologique chez le prématuré nouveau-né de mère traitée par Diazépam. J Gynécol Obstét Bio Reprod (Paris) 1973;2:357–366.
6 Autret E, Rey E, Laugier J, et al: Retentissement néonatal de la consommation de benzodiazépines au cours de la grossesse. Thérapie 1987;42:305–310.
7 Attallah A, Seilanian M, Bavoux F, et al: Psychotropes et grossesse. A propos de deux observations: Dosage du triazolam. Rev Fr Gynécol Obstét 1989;84:47–51.
8 Fisher JB, Edgren BE, Mammel MC, et al: Neonatal apnea associated with maternal clonazepam therapy: A case report. Obstet Gynecol 1985;66:34S–35S.
9 Morselli PL: Benzodiazepines; in: Drug Disposition during Development. New York, Spectrum Publications Halsed, 1977, pp 449–454.
10 Aun CST, Short SM, Leung DHY, et al: Induction dose-response of propofol in unpremedicated children. Br J Anaesth 1992;68:64–67.
11 Giese JL, Stockham RJ, Stanley TH, et al: Etomidate versus thiopental for induction of anesthesia. Anesth Analg 1985;64:871–876.
12 Morgan M, Lumley J, Whitwam JG: Etomidate: A new water-soluble non-barbiturate intravenous induction agent. Lancet 1975;i:955–956.
13 Jahangir SM, Rahman K: Prolonged apnoea, trismus and ketamine (letter). Anaesthesia 1991;46:1086.
14 Holden GG, Parsons JD: Severe respiratory depression and delayed recovery following the injection of diazepam and pentazocine. SAAD Dig 1981;4:280–282.
15 Hall AH, Smolinske SC, Conrad FL, et al: Ibuprofen overdose: 126 cases. Ann Emerg Med 1986;15:1308–1313.
16 Cooper GM, O'Connor M, Mark J, et al: Effect of alfentanil and fentanyl on recovery from brief anaesthesia. Br J Anaesthesiol 1983;55: 179S–182S.
17 Hickson GB, Altemeier WA, Martin ED, et al: Parental administration of chemical agents: A cause of apparent life-threatening events. Pediatrics 1989;83:772–776.
18 Naumburg EG, Meny RG: Breast milk opioids and neonatal apnea (letter). Am J Dis Child 1988;142: 11–12.
19 Billmire DA, Neale HW, Gregory RO: Use of IV fentanyl in the outpatient treatment of pediatric facial trauma. J Trauma 1985;25:1079–1080.
20 François C, Gouyon JB, Tenenbaum D, et al: Effets néonatals de la nalbuphine administrée au cours du travail. Arch Fr Pédiatr 1990;47: 763–765.
21 Stephen GW, Cooper LV, Harvey D: The effect of narcotic and narcotic-agonist drugs in the newborn rabbit. Br J Anaesth 1976;48:635–638.
22 Esener Z: Effect of fazadinium on respiratory functions and its correlation in neuromuscular transmission in children. Middle East J Anesthesiol 1987;9:97–107.
23 Benzer A, Luz G, Oswald E, et al: Succinylcholine induced prolonged apnea in a 3-week-old newborn: Treatment with human plasma cholinesterase. Anesth Analg 1992;74: 137–138.
24 Gill RS, O'Connell N, Scott RPF: Reversal of prolonged suxamethonium apnoea with fresh frozen plasma in a 6-week-old infant. Anaesthesia 1991;46:1036–1038.
25 Singer J, Janz T: Apnea and seizures caused by nicotine ingestion. Pediatr Emerg Care 1990;6:135–137.
26 Wenner D, Hamilton GC: Seizures following topical application of local anesthetics to burn patients. Ann Emerg Med 1984;13:456–458.
27 Webster AC, McKishnic JD, Kenyon CF, et al: Spinal anesthesia for inguinal hernia repair in high-risk neonates. Can J Anaesth 1991;38: 281–286.
28 Chasnof IJ, Hunt E, Kletter R, Kaplan D: Prenatal cocaine is associated with respiratory pattern abnormalities. AJDC 1989;143:583–587.
29 Chaney NE, Franke J, Wadlington WB: Cocaine convulsions in a breast-feeding baby. J Pediatr 1988; 112:134–135.
30 Yagupsky P, Gorodischer R: Massive clonidine ingestion with hypertension in a 9-month-old infant. Pediatrics 1983;72:500–502.
31 Artman M, Boerth RC: Clonidine poisoning, a complex problem. Am J Dis Child 1983;137:171–174.
32 Olson RJ, Bomberg BB, Zimmerman TJ: Apneic spells associated with timolol therapy in a neonate. Am J Ophthalmol 1979;88:120–122.
33 Hallidie-Smith KA: Prostaglandin E1 in suspected ductus dependent cardiac malformation. Arch Dis Child 1984;59:1020–1026.
34 Long W, Thompson T, Sundell H, et al: Effects of two rescue doses of a synthetic surfactant on mortality rate and survival without bronchopulmonary dysplasia in 700- to 1350-gram infants with respiratory distress syndrome. Pediatrics 1991; 118:595–605.

Biol Neonate 1994;65:258–264

Astrid Nehlig

INSERM U272,
Université de Nancy I,
Nancy, France

Effects of Respiratory Stimulants on Cerebral Metabolism and Blood Flow

Key Words

Respiratory stimulants
Methylxanthines
Caffeine
Theophylline
Aminophylline
Doxapram
Cerebral blood flow
Cerebral energy metabolism

Abstract

The cerebral metabolic and circulatory effects of the two main classes of respiratory stimulants used in the apnea of the newborn and premature infant, i.e. methylxanthines and doxapram, have not been studied in great detail. In adult animals and humans, methylxanthines widely increase cerebral metabolic rates and simultaneously decrease cerebral blood flow levels. Thus, these compounds are able to reset the level of coupling between cerebral blood flow and energy metabolism inducing a relative hypoperfusion at a constant metabolic rate. In neonates, methylxanthines induce no change in cerebral blood flow as long as the drop in pCO_2 related to drug administration is prevented. Information on doxapram effects on cerebral blood flow and metabolism is very scarse and limited to adult animals. Doxapram does not induce any change in cerebral energy metabolism and transiently decreases cerebral blood flow. In conclusion, it seems that the use of methylxanthines in apneic newborn infants fulfils a good margin of safety with respect to cerebral blood flow as long as no other pathology such as marked hypoxia or seizures is present. The use of doxapram also seems to stay in a good margin of safety in terms of cerebral blood flow and energy metabolism but many more studies are necessary to better understand the effects of this respiratory stimulant on cerebral functional activity.

Introduction

Methylxanthines (caffeine, theophylline, aminophylline) are frequently used as respiratory stimulants in both neonates to treat apnea of prematurity, bronchopulmonary displasia and in weaning infants the ventilator [1–6] as well as in adults to treat asthma [7]. Methylxanthines are well known stimulants of the central nervous system, resulting in increased alertness, wakefulness and activity [8]. The general increase in activity induced by methylxanthines translates into a stimulation in whole body metabolic rate as a result of both increased cellular metabolic activity and hyperventilation [9, 10]. Whereas adverse renal, cardiovascular and gastrointestinal side effects of methylxanthines have been identified [1, 2, 11], less information is available on the effects of these drugs on cerebral blood flow and metabolism [10].

Doxapram (1-ethyl-4-(2-morpholinoethyl)-3,3-2-pyrolidinone) is also used to stimulate respiration in both adults [12–14] and neo-

Astrid Nehlig
INSERM U272
Université de Nancy I
30, rue Lionnois, BP 3069
F–54013 Nancy Cedex (France)

0006–3126/94/
0654–0258$5.00/0

nates. In the latter case, doxapram is administered alone or associated to methylxanthines, mainly when apnea episodes persist in spite of caffeine treatment [15–19]. Doxapram has a wide convulsant to therapeutic ratio (70:1) [20, 21] and seems to act as a respiratory stimulant at least as efficient as caffeine and with less marked side effects than methylxanthines at doses regularly used in clinics [18, 22, 23]. Indeed, conversely to methylxanthines, doxapram does not induce any change in whole body metabolic rate [10]. Winnie [24] called doxapram the closest substance to a pure respirogenic agent. Compared to methylxanthines, even less is known on the effects of doxapram on cerebral blood flow (CBF) and energy metabolism [25].

In adults, methylxanthines reduce CBF [8] and several studies have suggested that events and therapeutic interventions that alter CBF in the preterm neonate may play a major role in the pathogenesis of intraventricular hemorrhage and periventricular leukomalacia [26, 27]. Therefore, it is important to keep in mind the effects of respiratory stimulants on CBF and metabolism especially to be able to remain in a margin of safety when using these drugs to treat apnea of prematurity.

Effects of Methylxanthines on Cerebral Blood Flow and Metabolism in Adults

Effects of Methylxanthines on Cerebral Energy Metabolism

The stimulant effects of caffeine on the cerebral nervous system are associated with changes in local rates of cerebral energy metabolism. Administration of an acute dose of 10 mg/kg caffeine or continuous perfusion of methylxanthine, at a rate of 0.30 mg/kg/min, induces an increase in the rates of local cerebral glucose utilization; this increase is significant in monoaminergic cell groupings, like substantia nigra and ventral tegmental area, which are rich in dopamine, medial and dorsal raphe nuclei, which contain serotonin and locus coeruleus, rich in noradrenaline. Caffeine also increases the rates of energy metabolism in the structures of the extrapyramidal motor system and in numerous thalamic nuclei and motor or limbic relays, as well as in limbic areas such as the hippocampus [28–34]. These local increases of cerebral glucose utilization in structures which are involved in the control of locomotor activity and especially in the sleep/wake cycle, correlate with the well-known methylxanthine-induced behavioral modifications. Finally, the increase in glucose utilization rates is of the same amplitude after acute or 2-week chronic administration of 10 mg/kg caffeine. Thus, cerebral energy metabolism does not seem to develop tolerance to the stimulant effects of methylxanthine [29].

Effects of Methylxanthines on Cerebral Blood Flow

Methylxanthines such as caffeine or theophylline induce vasodilation, except in the central nervous system where they raise cerebrovascular resistance; this actually contributes to a reduction in CBF. The cerebral vasoconstrictive properties of methylxanthines have been demonstrated in both humans [35–43] and animals [32–34, 44, 45]. Caffeine induces a decrease in local CBF, mainly in the areas where it increases metabolism, i.e. in monoaminergic cell groupings, in the motor and limbic systems, and in the thalamus [33, 34, 44].

Coupling between Cerebral Blood Flow and Metabolism

In most situations, CBF and glucose utilization are closely coupled in all cerebral regions [46–49], so that modifications in cerebral activity elicit parallel changes in glucose utilization and in CBF [49–53]. In general, changes in CBF are the consequence of variations in cerebral energy metabolism [50, 52, 53]. Contrary to the majority of pharmacological agents to which man is frequently exposed, caffeine has the property of inducing cerebral hypoperfusion accompanied by simultaneous increase in glucose utilization [28–34, 44]; in other words, it resets the level of coupling between CBF and energy metabolism. Methylxanthines thus seem to modify the regulating mechanism between CBF and cerebral metabolism. Although this mechanism is not yet well understood, adenosine, with which methylxanthines compete, is known to be one of the modulators of regulation in the relationship of blood flow to metabolism in the central nervous system [51, 54, 55].

Effects of Methylxanthines on Cerebral Blood Flow and Metabolism in Newborns

Methylxanthines are very frequently used in the treatment of idiopathic apnea in the preterm infant [1–4, 6]. The effects of methylxanthines on cerebral energy metabolism in premature and newborn infants have not been investigated in detail. Only one study reports increases in cerebral metabolic rate after administration of aminophylline in young mice [56].

More data are available on the effects of these drugs on CBF. Some authors reported reduction in CBF up to 21% after administration of 6–10 mg/kg theophylline or aminophylline in newborn [57] and premature infants [58–60]. The latter study shows, however, that the decrease in CBF velocity, assessed by Doppler ultrasonography, is not accompanied by adverse effects on cerebral function (visual evoked potentials) in stable, preterm infants [60]. Conversely, many other studies show that CBF velocity is not affected by methylxanthines, even at the quite high common loading dose of 20 mg/kg caffeine used to treat apnea in preterm infants [61–64]. However, it appears important to maintain the level of arterial pCO_2 in the physiological range, since it is not known whether the decrease in CBF is directly related to the methylxanthine administration or secondary to the decrease in arterial pCO_2 induced by the drug [65]. Indeed, hypocapnia has been recorded after methylxanthine administration in both preterm neonates [60, 66] and in adult animals [28–32] and humans [35]. The decrease in CBF can be avoided and thus methylxanthine safely used in the treatment of apnea of prematurity when pCO_2 is monitored and maintained at a constant level [67].

Effects of Methylxanthines on Cerebral Blood Flow in Pathological States

In adult rats, rabbits and dogs, theophylline has been shown to significantly attenuate or even block the increase in CBF recorded during moderate and severe hypoxia [68–72], whereas the methylxanthine does not influence either cerebral hypoxic hyperemia at the level of cerebrocortical microcirculation in adult cats [73] or hypoxia-induced increase in CBF in newborn piglets [74]. Moreover, theophylline produces no significant effect on hypercapnia-induced increase in CBF [68, 69]. These results confirm the specificity of action of theophylline and other methylxanthines on hypoxia-induced adenosine release [68–72, 75] and do not support a role for adenosine as a mediator of cerebral hypoxic hyperemia in the newborn piglet [74]. However, the latter data on changes induced by methylxanthines in neonatal CBF rates during hypoxia need further exploration. Likewise, theophylline significantly reduces the hyperemia observed during seizures in adult animals, prevents tissue hyperoxia and enhances brain damage. These data strongly suggest that adenosine is partly responsible for the increase in CBF recorded during seizures and has neuroprotective effects [76].

Taken together, these data seem to reassure the safety of methylxanthine treatment with respect to CBF in stable, apneic infants. However, in sick premature or newborn infants, the use of methylxanthine may be more questionable.

Effects of Doxapram on Cerebral Blood Flow and Metabolism

There are only very few studies available on the effects of doxapram on cerebral energy metabolism and blood flow. Moreover, information on the effects of the respiratory stimulant of the parameters of brain functional activity in neonates are totally lacking.

Effects of Doxapram on Cerebral Energy Metabolism

In adult rats, an infusion of doxapram at doses inducing circulating levels of the drug of the same order of magnitude as those recorded in human neonates treated with the respiratory stimulant does not significant changes in the levels of cerebral energy metabolism [77, 78]. These data confirm the absence of side effects of doxapram compared to methylxanthines when used as respiratory stimulants. They are also in favor of a preferentially central or mixed central and peripheral action of methylxanthines on respiration and a more peripheral action of doxapram on chemoreceptors, at least at therapeutic levels [77, 78].

Effect of Doxapram on Cerebral Blood Flow

As for energy metabolism, the effects of doxapram have only been studied in adult animals. In anesthetized and unanesthetized goats, a central injection of doxapram via the temporal artery, in doses too small to affect peripheral circulation, produces an immediate and prolonged decrease in CBF which is not related to changes in arterial pCO_2. These data indicate that doxapram constricts the cerebral vasculature in a way unrelated to changes in blood gases and peripheral hemodynamics [79]. When doxapram is given in clinical doses by peripheral i.v. injection to anesthetized and unanesthetized goats, the drug produces a biphasic response. CBF, cardiac output, blood pressure and heart rate decrease abruptly, but, with the exception of CBF, return to or exceed preinjection values within 30 s. CBF returns to preinjection values within 10 min and stays stable in animals ventilated with 100% O_2 whereas CBF continues to increase and reaches a peak at 20 min in animals breathing room air [79]. These changes are not secondary to changes in blood gases, contrarily to previous data showing that doxapram-induced changes in CBF are a consequence of the effects of the drug on respiration and blood gases [80].

The effects of doxapram on CBF were also evaluated in a group of adult rats with intracranial hypertension since the main cause of sudden death in that kind of patients is respiratory failure. The administration of 10 mg/kg of doxapram to some of these animals improved the respiratory condition and increased cerebral perfusion pressure and regional CBF [81]. Obviously, more investigation is required to understand the cerebral hemodynamic effects of doxapram in both control and sick animals as well as its effects on CBF and energy metabolism in neonates.

In summary, these few data seem to confirm the good margin of safety of doxapram with respect to cerebral functional activity, as pointed out previously [20, 21].

Conclusion

In conclusion, it appears that, in adult humans and animals, methylxanthines widely increase cerebral energy metabolism and decrease CBF. These substances are thus able to reset the level of coupling between CBF and energy metabolism inducing a relative hypoperfusion of the brain at a constant metabolic level. However, the effects of methylxanthines on cerebral functional activity are accompanied by a decrease in arterial pCO_2. Indeed, in human neonates, methylxanthines do not decrease CBF when the drop in pCO_2 is prevented. Conversely, doxapram has no effect on cerebral glucose utilization and only transiently decreases CBF in adult animals.

Taken together, the available data suggest that, at the doses regularly used in clinics, both methylxanthines and doxapram may have a quite good margin of safety with respect to CBF and brain energy metabolism in human neonates suffering from apnea. However, data on the effects of methylxanthines and doxapram on cerebral energy metabolism and blood flow in newborn animals and humans are still lacking. We are therefore in need to define an animal model closer than the rat to the human brain which would allow the measurement of both cerebral functional activity in the neonate and the effects of respiratory stimulants on cerebral metabolism and blood flow.

Acknowledgements

The author wishes to thank C. Creusat for editorial assistance.

References

1 Aranda JV, Grondin D, Sasyniuk BI: Pharmacologic considerations in the therapy of neonatal apnea. Pediatr Clin North Am 1981;28:113–133.
2 Aranda JV, Turmen T: Methylxanthines in apnea of prematurity. Clin Perinatol 1979:6:87–109.
3 Bairam A, Boutroy MJ, Badonnel Y, Vert P: Theophylline versus caffeine: Comparative effects in treatment of idiopathic apnea in the preterm infant. J Pediatr 1987;4:636–639.
4 Bednarek FJ, Roloff DW: Treatment of apnea of prematurity with aminophylline. Pediatrics 1976;58: 335–339.
5 Rooklin AR, Moomjian AS, Shutack JG, et al: Theophylline therapy in bronchopulmonary dysplasia. J Pediatr 1979;95:882–885.
6 Shannon DC, Gotay F, Stein IM, et al: Prevention of apnea and bradycardia in low-birthweight infants. Pediatrics 1975;55:589–594.
7 Rall TW: Drugs used in the treatment of asthma. The methylxanthines, cromolyn sodium and other agents; in Goodman A, Gilman P, Rall TW, Nies AS, Taylor P (eds): The Pharmacological Basis of Therapeutics. New York, Pergamon, 1990, pp 618–637.
8 Vonlanthen MG, McCarter RJ, Casto DT: Metabolic effects of aminophylline in rats. Am J Physiol 1989; 256:R1274–R1278.
9 Côté A, Blanchard P, Meehan B: Metabolic and cardiorespiratory effects of doxapram and theophylline in sleeping newborn piglets. J Appl Physiol 1992;72:410–415.
10 Nehlig A, Daval JL, Debry G: Caffeine and the central nervous system: Mechanisms of action, biochemical, metabolic and psychostimulant effects. Brain Res Rev 1992; in press.
11 Zakauddin S, Leake RD, Trygstad CW: Theophylline increases glomerular filtration rate in preterm infants. Dev Pharmacol Ther 1980;1: 333–338.
12 Moser KM, Luchsinger PC, Adamson JS, et al: Respiratory stimulation with intravenous doxapram in respiratory failure. A double-blind co-operative study. N Engl J Med 1973;288:427–431.
13 Lareng L, Vaysse C, Cathala B: Use of doxapram hydrochloride in the treatment of drug induced toxic comas. Can J Anaesth 1971;19:1059–1072.
14 Allen CJ, Gough KR: Effect of doxapram on heavy sedation produced by intravenous diazepam. Br Med J 1983;286:1181–1182.
15 Burnard ED, Moore RG, Nichol H: A trial of doxapram in the recurrent apnea of prematurity; in Stern L, Oh W, Friis-Hansen B (eds): Intensive Care in the Newborn, part II. New York, Masson, 1978, pp 43–148.

16 Alpan G, Eyal F, Sagi E, et al: Doxapram in the treatment of idiopathic apnea of prematurity unresponsive to aminophylline. J Pediatr 1984; 104:634–637.
17 Barrington KJ, Finer NN, Torok-Both G, et al: Dose-response relationship of doxapram in the therapy for refractory idiopathic apnea of prematurity. Pediatrics 1987;80:22–27.
18 Bairam A, Vert P: Low-dose doxapram for apnea of prematurity. Lancet 1986;i:793–794.
19 Peliowski A, Finer NN: A blinded, randomized placebo-controlled trial to compare theophylline and doxapram for the treatment of apnea of prematurity. J Pediatr 1990;116: 648-653.
20 Funderburk WH, Alphine RS: Electrical changes in the CNS produced by a new respiratory stimulant, AHR 619. Fed Proc 1962;21:324.
21 Ward JW, Franko BV: A new centrally acting agent (AHR-619) with marked respiratory stimulation, pressor, and 'awakening' effects. Fed Proc 1962;21:325.
22 Baxter AD: Side effects of doxapram infusion. Eur J Intens Care Med 1976;2:87–88.
23 Hayakawa F, Hakamada S, Kuno K, et al: Doxapram in the treatment of idiopathic apnea of prematurity: Desirable dosage and serum concentrations. J Pediatr 1986;109:138–140.
24 Winnie AP: Chemical respirogenesis: A comparative study. Acta Anaesth Scand 1973;51(suppl):2–32.
25 Bairam A, Boutroy MJ, Vert P: Un stimulant respiratoire, le doxapram, et ses applications en pédiatrie. Arch Fr Pédiatr 1992;49:469–474.
26 Ment LR, Ehrenkranz RA, Lange RC: Alterations in cerebral blood in preterm infants with intraventricular hemorrhage. Pediatrics 1981;68: 763–769.
27 Levene M, Fawer C, Lamont R: Risk factors in the development of intraventricular hemorrhage in the preterm neonate. Arch Dis Child 1982;57:410–417.
28 Nehlig A, Lucignani G, Kadekaro M, et al: Effects of acute administration of caffeine on local cerebral glucose utilization in the rat. Eur J Pharmacol 1984;101:91–100.
29 Nehlig A, Daval JL, Boyet S, Vert P: Comparative effects of acute and chronic administration of caffeine on local cerebral glucose utilization in the conscious rat. Eur J Pharmacol 1986;129:933–103.
30 Nehlig A, Pereira de Vasconcelos A, Boyet S, Vert P: Influence d'une administration chronique et aiguë de caféine sur l'utilisation cérébrale locale de glucose et sur l'activité locomotrice du rat. Circ Métab Cerveau 1987;4:67–79.
31 Nehlig A, Pereira de Vasconcelos A, Collignon A, Boyet S: Comparative effects of caffeine and L-phenylisopropyladenosine on local cerebral glucose utilization in the rat. Eur J Pharmacol 1988;157:1–11.
32 Nehlig A, Dumont I, Pereira de Vasconcelos A, Boyet S: Influence de l'administration de caféine et/ou de L-phénylisopropyladénosine sur l'activité locomotrice et le couplage entre le débit sanguin et le métabolisme cérébral chez le rat. Circ Métab Cerveau 1990;7:99–116.
33 Grome JJ, Stefanovich V: Differential effects of xanthine derivatives on local cerebral blood flow and glucose utilization in the conscious rat; in Stefanovich V, Rudolphi K, Schubert P (eds): Adenosine: Receptors and Modulation of Cell Function. Oxford, IRL Press, 1985, pp 453–457.
34 Grome JJ, Stefanovich V: Differential effects of methylxanthines on local cerebral blood flow and glucose utilization in the conscious rat. Naunyn-Schmiedeberg's Arch Pharmacol 1986;333:172–177.
35 Wechsler RL, Kleiss LM, Kety SS: The effects of intravenously administered aminophylline on cerebral circulation and metabolism in man. J Clin Invest 1950;29:28–30.
36 Shenkin HA: Effects of various drugs upon cerebral circulation and metabolism in man. J Appl Physiol 1951;3:465–471.
37 Moyer JH, Tashnek AB, Miller SJ, et al: The effect of theophylline with ethylene diamine (aminophylline) and caffeine on cerebral hemodynamics and cerebral fluid pressure in patients with hypertensive headache. Am J Med Sci 1952;224:377–385.
38 Gottstein U, Paulson OB: The effects of intracarotid aminophylline on the cerebral circulation. Stroke 1972;3:560–565.
39 Magnussen I, Hoedt-Rasmussen K: The effect of intraarterial administered aminophylline on cerebral hemodynamics in man. Acta Neurol Scand 1977;55:131–136.
40 Mathew RJ, Barr DL, Weinman ML: Caffeine and cerebral blood flow. Br J Psychiatry 1983;143:604–608.
41 Mathew RJ, Wilson WH: Caffeine induced changes in cerebral circulation. Stroke 1985;16:814–817.
42 Cameron OG, Modell JG, Hariharan M: Caffeine and human cerebral blood flow: A positron emission tomography study. Life Ssi 1990;47: 1141–1146.
43 Mathew RJ, Wilson WH: Behavioral and cerebrovascular effects of caffeine in patients with anxiety disorders. Acta Psychiatr Scand 1990;82: 17–22.
44 Nehlig A, Pereira de Vasconcelos A, Dumont I, Boyet S: Effects of caffeine, *L*-phenylisopropyladenosine and their combination on local cerebral blood flow in the rat. Eur J Pharmacol 1990;179:271–280.
45 Puiroud S, Pinard E, Seylaz J: Dynamic cerebral and systemic circulatory effects of adenosine, theophylline and dipyridamole. Brain Res 1988;453:287–298.
46 Des Rosiers MH, Kennedy C, Patlak CS, et al: Relationship between local cerebral blood flow and glucose utilization in the rat. Neurology 1974;24:389.
47 Reivich M: Blood flow metabolism couple; in Plum F (ed): Brain Dysfunction in Metabolic Disorders. New York, Raven Press, 1974, pp 125–140.
48 Raichle ME, Herscovitch P, Mintun MA: Dynamic measurements of local cerebral blood flow and metabolism using positron emission tomography; in Greitz T, Ingvar DH, Widen L (eds): The Metabolism of the Human Brain Studied with Positron Emission Tomography. New York, Raven Press, 1985, pp 159–164.

49 Sokoloff L: Local cerebral energy metabolism: its relationship to local functional activity and blood flow; in Purves MJ, Elliott K (eds): Cerebral Vascular Smooth Muscle and Its Control. Amsterdam, Elsevier/ Excerpta Medica/North Holland, 1978, pp 171–197.
50 Kelly PAT, McCulloch J: The effect of GABAergic agonist muscimol upon the relationship between cerebral blood flow and glucose utilization. Brain Res 1983;258:338–342.
51 Kuschinsky W: Coupling between functional metabolism and blood flow in the brain. State of the art. Microcirculation 1983;2:357–378.
52 McCulloch J, Kelly PAT, Ford I: Effect of apomorphine on the relationship between local cerebral glucose utilization and local cerebral blood flow (with an appendix on its statistical analysis). J Cereb Blood Flow Metab 1982;2:487–499.
53 Grome JJ, Harper AM: The effects of quipazone: A putative serotonin agonist on local cerebral blood flow and glucose utilization in the rat, and pial vascular diameter in the cat. J Cereb Blood Flow Metab 1983;3(suppl):S302–S303.
54 Berne RM, Winn RH, Rubio R: The local regulation of cerebral blood flow. Prog Cerebrovasc Dis 1981; 24:243–260.
55 Winn HR, Rubio R, Berne RM: The role of adenosine in the regulation of cerebral blood flow. J Cereb Blood Flow Metab 1981;1:239–244.
56 Thurston JH, Hauhart RE, Dirgo JA: Aminophylline increases cerebral metabolic rate and decreases anoxic survival in young mice. Science 1978;201:649–651.
57 Friis-Hansen B: Cerebral blood flow in the newborn infant. Cardiovascular and respiratory physiology in the fetus and neonates. Coll INSERM 1986;95–108.
58 Rosenkrantz TS, Oh W: Aminophylline reduces cerebral blood flow velocity in low-birth-weight infants. Am J Dis Child 1984;138:489–491.
59 McDonnell M, Ives NK, Hope PL: Intravenous aminophylline and cerebral blood flow in preterm infants. Arch Dis Child 1992;67:416–418.
60 Pryds O, Schneider S: Aminophylline reduces cerebral blood flow in stable, preterm infants without affecting the visual evoked potential. Eur J Pediatr 1991;150:366–369.
61 Ghai V, Raju TNK, Kim SY, McCulloch K: Regional cerebral blood flow velocity after aminophylline therapy in premature newborn infants. J Pediatr 1989;5:870–873.
62 Saliba E, Autret E, Gold F: Caffeine and cerebral blood flow velocity in preterm infants. Dev Pharmacol Ther 1989;13:134–138.
63 Saliba E, Autret E, Gold F, et al: Effect of caffeine on cerebral blood flow velocity in preterm infants. Biol Neonate 1989;56:198–203.
64 Van Bel F, Van de Bor M, Stijnen T, et al: Does caffeine affect cerebral blood flow in the preterm infants? Acta Pediatr Scand 1989;78:205–209.
65 Gottstein U, Held K, Sebening H, Steiner K: Is decrease of cerebral blood flow after intravenous injections of theophylline due to direct vasoconstrictive action of the drug? Eur Neurol 1971/72;6:153–157.
66 Davi MJ, Sankaran K, Simons KJ, et al: Physiologic changes induced by theophylline in the treatment of apnea in preterm infants. J Pediatr 1978;92:91–95.
67 Sonestreet BS, Nowicki PT, Hansen NB, et al: Effect of aminophylline on brain blood flow in the newborn piglet. Dev Pharmacol Ther 1973;6: 248–258.
68 Emerson TE Jr, Raymond RM: Involvement of adenosine in cerebral hypoxic hyperemia in the dog. Am J Physiol 1981;241:H134–H138.
69 Hoffman WE, Albrecht RF, Miletich DJ: The role of adenosine in CBF increases during hypoxia in young vs. aged rats. Stroke 1984;15: 124–129.
70 Morii S, Winn HR, Berne RM: Effect of theophylline, an adenosine receptor blocker, on cerebral blood flow (CBF) during rest and transient hypoxia. J Cereb Blood Flow Metab 1981;3(suppl 1):S480–S481.
71 Morii S, Ngai AC, Ko KR, Winn HR: Role of adenosine in regulation of cerebral blood flow: Effects of theophylline during normoxia and hypoxia. Am J Physiol 1987;253: H165–H175.
72 Pinard E, Puiroud S, Seylaz J: Role of adenosine in cerebral hypoxic hyperemia in the unanesthetized rabbit. Brain Res 1989;481:124–130.
73 Dora E: Effect of theophylline treatment on the functional hyperaemic and hypoxic responses of cerebrocortical microcirculation. Acta Physiol Hung 1986;68:183–197.
74 McPhee AJ, Maxwell GM: The effect of theophylline on regional cerebral blood flow responses to hypoxia in newborn piglets. Pediatr Res 1987;6:573–578.
75 Wahl M, Kuschinsky W: The dilatory action of adenosine on pial arterioles of cats and its inhibition by theophylline. Pflügers Arch 1976;362: 55–59.
76 Pinard E, Riche D, Puiroud S, Seylaz J: Theophylline reduces cerebral hyperemia and enhances brain damage induced by seizures. Brain Res 1990;511:303–309.
77 Schroeder H, Boyet S, Nehlig A: Effects of caffeine and doxapram perfusion on local cerebral glucose utilization in conscious rats. Eur J Pharmacol 1989;167:245–254.
78 Schroeder H, Boyet S, Nehlig A: Effects de l'administration de cafèine et de doxapram sur l'utilisation cérébrale locale de glucose chez le rat. Circ Métab Cerveau 1989;6:160–173.
79 Miletich DJ, Ivankovich AD, Albrecht RF, et al: The effects of doxapram on cerebral blood flow and peripheral hemodynamics in the anesthetized and unanesthetized goat. Anesth Analg 1976;55:279–285.
80 Funderburk WH, Oliver KL, Ward JW: Modification of cerebral blood flow in dogs with doxapram hydrochloride. Toxicol Appl Pharmacol 1968;13:67–75.
81 Namba H, Akimoto M, Yamaura A, et al: Effects of a respiratory stimulant on intracranial pressure and cerebral blood flow. Neurol Med Chir (Tokyo) 1983;23:515–520.

Biol Neonate 1994;65:265–271

Robert T. Brouillette[a]
Mirella Marzocchi[b]

[a] Department of Pediatrics, Montreal Children's Hospital and McGill University, Montreal, Canada;
[b] Department of Pediatrics, Northwestern University, Chicago, Ill., USA

Diaphragm Pacing: Clinical and Experimental Results

Key Words

Central hypoventilation syndrome
Artificial respiration
Muscle transformation
Diaphragmatic pacing
Breathing children

Abstract

Over the last 26 years diaphragm pacing has been used in over 400 adults and 70 children to support ventilation and oxygenation. Diaphragm pacing can be useful for conditions in which the brain stem respiratory centers provide little or no stimulation to the respiratory muscles, i.e. central hypoventilation syndrome, Arnold-Chiari malformation/brain stem dysfunction, and high quadriplegia. Because the pacing systems are so portable, the greatest advantages accrue to those patients who require ventilatory support both while awake and asleep. Infants and children require tracheostomy to avoid upper airway obstruction and bilateral pacing to meet higher metabolic demands. The stimulus parameters most appropriate for pediatric patients have been characterized as low stimulus frequency, short inspiratory time, and moderate respiratory rate. Use of similar stimulus parameters in an immature animal model has resulted in preservation of diaphragmatic structure and function but transformation of the diaphragm from a mixed muscle to one with a uniform population of type 1, fatigue-resistant fibers (physiologic, histochemical, myosin isoform, and ultrastructural evidence). In 33 pediatric patients, representing 96 patient-years of use, there were 26 failures of the pacing systems requiring removal and/or replacement of the internal components. Mean time to failure was 56 months. Of our 36 patients who had diaphragm pacing systems implanted, 26 are alive and 22 are currently using the pacing systems. Two recent advances may further improve the long-term outcome of patients using diaphragm pacing. Smaller, better encapsulated receivers may improve system longevity and a new stimulus electrode may reduce the risk of diaphragmatic damage.

History

The clinical use of electrical stimulation of the phrenic nerves was begun by Sarnoff et al. [1] in 1948–1951. Although they supported breathing for up to 3.5 days, the first long-term support of breathing awaited the development of a radiofrequency powered, partially implantable system. In 1964, Glenn et al. [2] began using this system in adults to pro-

Robert T. Brouillette, MD
Montreal Children's Hospital
Room C-920
2300, Tupper Street
Montreal, PQ H3H 1P3 (Canada)

0006–3126/94/
0654–0265$5.00/0

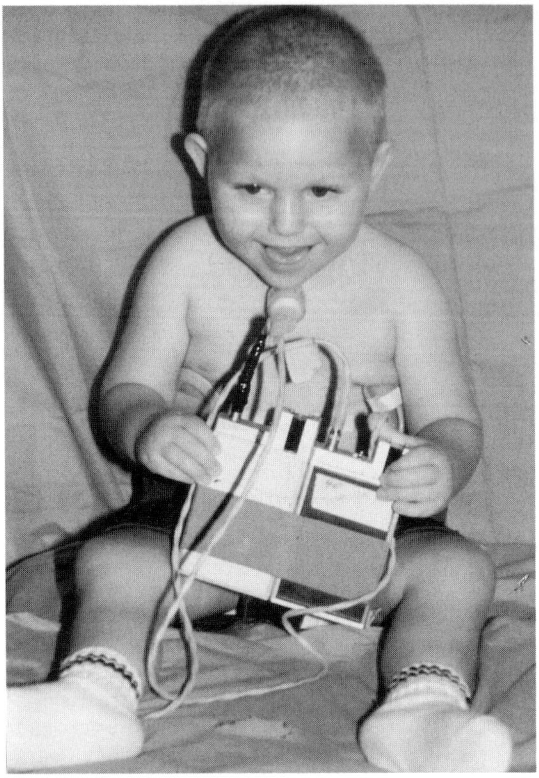

Fig. 1. A young boy with severe idiopathic congenital central hypoventilation syndrome using diaphragm pacing. Spontaneous ventilation was inadequate both during wakefulness and sleep. Ventilation has been supported using diaphragm pacing during wakefulness and a home positive pressure ventilator during sleep.

vide breathing support to high quadriplegics and patients with absent or inadequate spontaneous respiratory drive. In 1970, Mellins et al. [3] first reported a case of congenital central hypoventilation. Since 1976, diaphragm pacing has been used by Hunt and co-workers [4–6] in Chicago, as well as other centers, to support breathing in infants and children with central hypoventilation syndrome, high quadriplegia, and Arnold-Chiari malformation.

The current paper will review clinical aspects of this technology in infants and children and provide experimental animal data demonstrating the types of changes occurring in the diaphragm of immature mammals subjected to long-term diaphragm stimulation.

Diaphragm Pacing Systems

There are currently two approved systems for diaphragm pacing (Avery Laboratories Inc., Glen Cove, N.Y., USA; Atrostim, Tampere, Finland). We have used the first of these systems (fig. 1). The system consists of four components: an external radiofrequency transmitter, an external transmitting antenna, an implanted receiver which converts the radiofrequency signal to an electrical current, and a stimulating electrode on the phrenic nerve. Avery's newest system features a smaller receiver thought to have a longer functional life. A new digital system from Finland (Atrostim) uses a system of four stimulating electrodes, and has three switch-selectable settings for level of stimulation.

Indications and Diagnoses

Whereas in adults the most common indication for diaphragm pacing (DP) has been high quadriplegia, most children have had central hypoventilation syndrome [2, 5]. The Chicago group has now implanted 36 pacers in infants and children since 1976 for the following indications: congenital central hypoventilation syndrome (CHS), 25; childhood onset CHS, 2; CHS due to Arnold-Chiari malformation, 3; acquired hypoventilation, 1; and high quadriplegia, 5 [7]. Central hypoventilation syndrome is characterized by severely impaired ventilation, and ventilatory and arousal responses during quiet sleep [3–5]. In more severe cases ventilation is inadequate during wakefulness as well as sleep [7]. Spontaneous tidal volumes are typically too

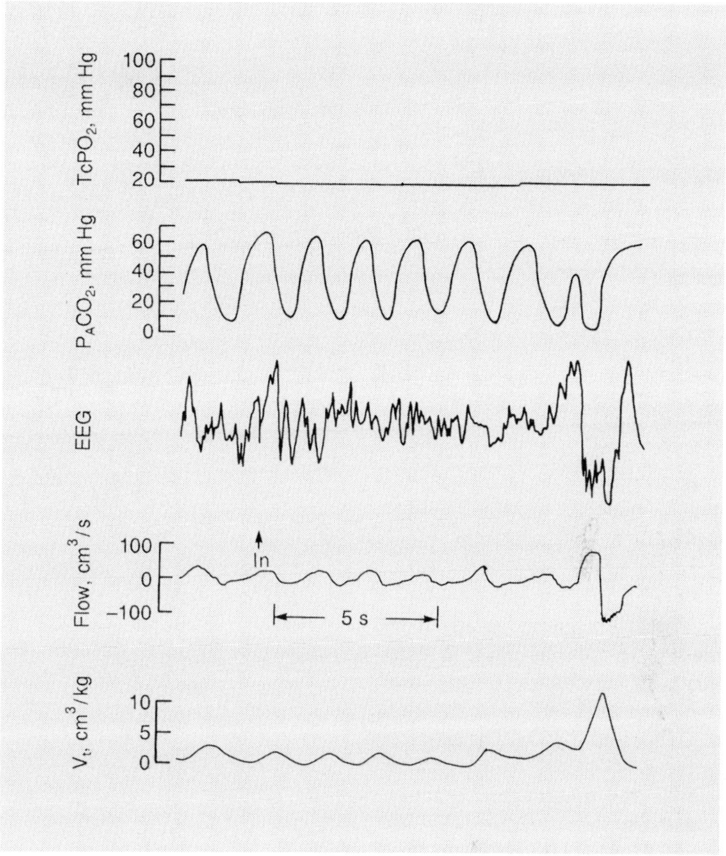

Fig. 2. Polygraphic tracing. Breathing abnormalities during sleep in a patient with central hypoventilation. Note the marked hypoxemia and hypercapnia. Tidal volumes (V_t) of approximately 3 cm^3/kg body weight were only slightly above anatomical dead space. The large breath at the end of the trace accompanied an arousal from sleep. T_cPO_2 = Transcutaneous partial pressure of oxygen; P_ACO_2 = end-tidal partial pressure of carbon dioxide; EEG = electroencephalogram; IN = inspiration. From Ilbawi et al. [8].

small to provide effective gas exchange (fig. 2). Diaphragm pacing establishes adequate alveolar ventilation eliminating hypoxemia and hypercarbia (fig. 3).

Selection of Patients

Selection of children for diaphragm pacing requires experience and careful consideration of medical and psychosocial factors. The responsible physician should be able to answer the following questions before proceeding with diaphragm pacing. Are the phrenic nerves, diaphragms, and lungs normal or nearly so? Will use of diaphragm pacing significantly improve the patient's quality of life? Usually, such improvement relates to improved mobility with diaphragm pacing compared to positive pressure ventilation. Do the benefits outweigh the risks of perioperative complications, possible phrenic nerve damage, infection, and system failure? Is there a comprehensive team available to provide for all aspects of care? Finally, will the child be discharged to a supportive family that will be able to assure that the benefits of diaphragm pacing accrue to their child?

Infants and children require several special considerations. Both diaphragms must be paced simultaneously to achieve adequate tidal volumes and tracheostomy is always re-

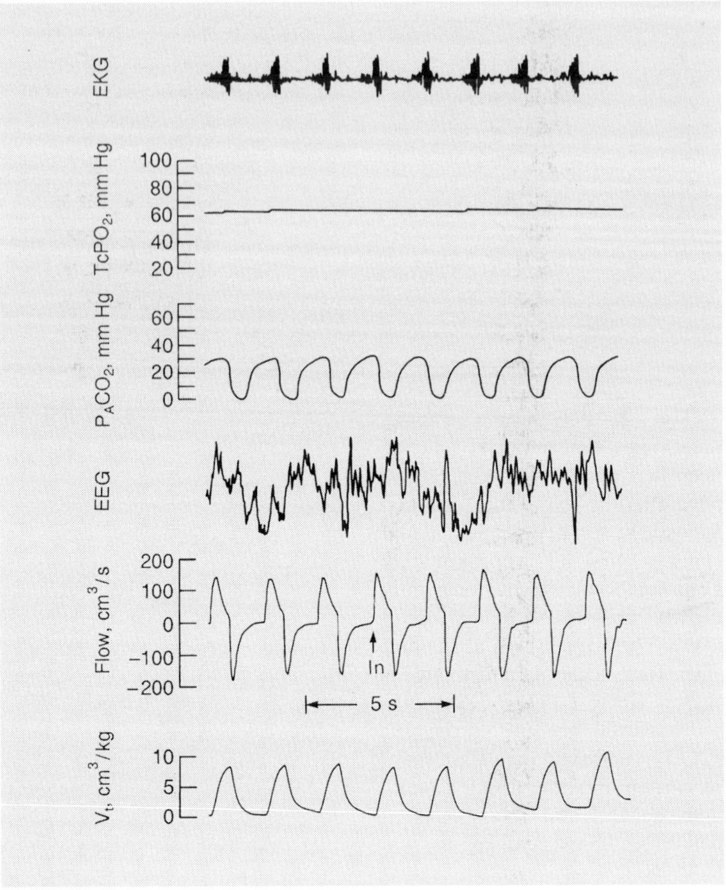

Fig. 3. Polygraph tracing from the same patient as figure 2. Adequate gas exchange during diaphragm pacing with normalization of $TcPO_2$ and P_ACO_2. The artifacts in the EKG signal are pacemaker stimuli and diaphragmatic action potentials. Tidal volumes (V_t) are approximately 9 ml/kg. From Ilbawi et al. [8].

quired. We prefer to wait until an infant is at least 6–12 months old before beginning diaphragm pacing. Intrathoracic electrode placement is preferred. Because the greatest benefit of diaphragm pacing is increased mobility, it is important to know if spontaneous awake ventilation is adequate. If awake ventilation is inadequate (fig. 1) pacers may be used during the day and a ventilator may be used at night. If awake ventilation is adequate, there may be less benefit as a portable ventilator may provide adequate ventilation during sleep when mobility is not an issue.

Outcomes for 36 patients implanted by the Chicago group were recently summarized [7]. Ten of 36 (28%) patients had died and another 4 (11%) were not using diaphragm pacing. Four deaths early in the series were related to overuse of diaphragm pacing when other backup systems were not available. Two deaths may have been related to the unrecognized development of an awake ventilatory deficiency and cor pulmonale [7]. Two potentially preventable deaths in unmonitored patients stress the need to monitor these patients whenever a caretaker is not in attendance. As standard apnea monitors do not detect airway obstruction, pulse oximetry or end-tidal CO_2 monitoring is preferred [9].

Pacemaker System Failures

The most common reason for the diaphragm pacing system to fail is a broken antenna. Unlike external components that can easily be replaced, replacement of internal components requires reoperation. In 33 children and 96 patient-years we found a mean time to failure of 4 years and 8 months [10]. Receiver failures [15] were followed by electrode wire breakage [6] and infection [3] as the causes necessitating reoperation. In 2 cases mechanical injury to the phrenic nerve was caused by the diaphragm pacing electrode. We anticipate fewer reoperations with improved receiver design and operative technique.

Imaging

Prior to implanting diaphragm pacers, the brain and cervical spinal cord should be visualized using magnetic resonance imaging (MRI) [11]. Although the brain stem is usually normal in idiopathic central hypoventilation syndrome (CHS) cortical atrophy is frequently seen. In our series, 2 of 5 patients with Arnold-Chiari malformation and CHS had treatable lesions – hindbrain compression and syringobulbia, respectively. We have seen one infant and one child with brain stem tumors causing CHS. Once diaphragm pacers are inserted, an MRI cannot be obtained.

Pacemaker Adjustments

The pacemaker should be adjusted to maintain adequate gas exchange while minimizing stimulus current [5]. Glenn et al. [12] developed the technique of low-frequency pacing allowing 24 h/day support of ventilation without diaphragmatic fatigue or damage [12]. We subsequently adapted this strategy for pediatric patients finding a low frequency, short inspiratory time and moderate respiratory rate most desirable [6]. However, 24 h/day pacing should not be considered routine for infants and children [5–7].

Animal Studies and Implications for Pediatric Patients

Work by Glenn's group showed that long-term low-frequency diaphragm pacing had important effects on the diaphragm of adults and mature mammals. No adverse effects were seen on the phrenic nerves but the diaphragm muscle changed from a mixture of type I and type II fibers to a homogeneous population of type I fibers [12–15]. In quadriplegics low-frequency pacing improved the strength of the atrophic diaphragm [12]. No data were available for immature mammals. Therefore, we examined the functional and structural effects of continuous low-frequency diaphragm pacing on the left hemidiaphragm of 5 immature dogs aged 65 ± 2 (SD) days at onset of pacing [16]. Stimulus parameters approximated those required to pace infants: stimulus frequency 11.1 Hz, inspiratory time 810 ms, and respiratory rate 20 breaths/min. Animals were paced 24 h/day for 24–28 days. Paced tidal volumes and airway occlusion pressures were unchanged at low (<15 Hz) stimulus frequencies but were reduced at high (>20 Hz) stimulus frequencies (fig. 4). Although histologically the paced hemidiaphragms appeared normal, histochemical studies showed a conversion from a mixture of type I (54%) and type II (46%) fibers to a uniform population of type I fibers with high oxidative enzyme activity (fig. 5). Transformation of muscle type was also demonstrated by pyrophosphate gel electrophoresis; fast and slow isomyosin bands were noted in control specimens, whereas only slow isomyosin was

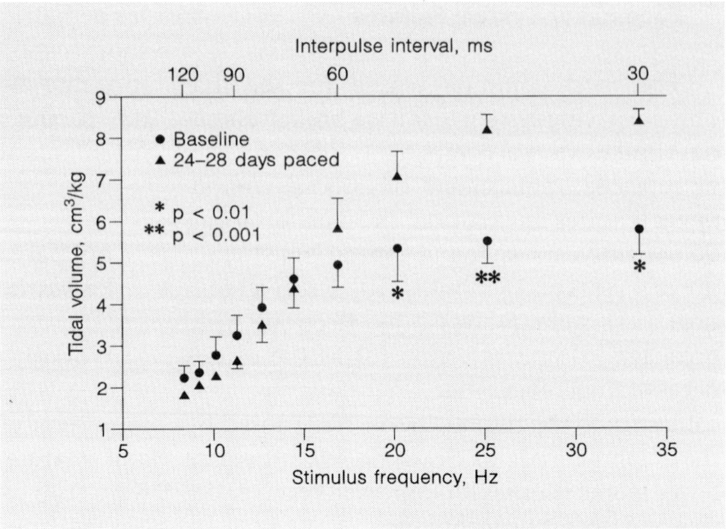

Fig. 4. Paced tidal volumes (mean ± SEM of 5 animals) at various stimulus frequencies from 8.3 to 33 Hz (interpulse intervals 120–30 ms). Values before and after 24–28 days of continuous low-frequency pacing are shown. Note the preservation of tidal volumes at low and moderate stimulus frequencies and the decrease in tidal volumes after pacing at stimulus frequencies above 20 Hz. From Marzocchi et al. [16].

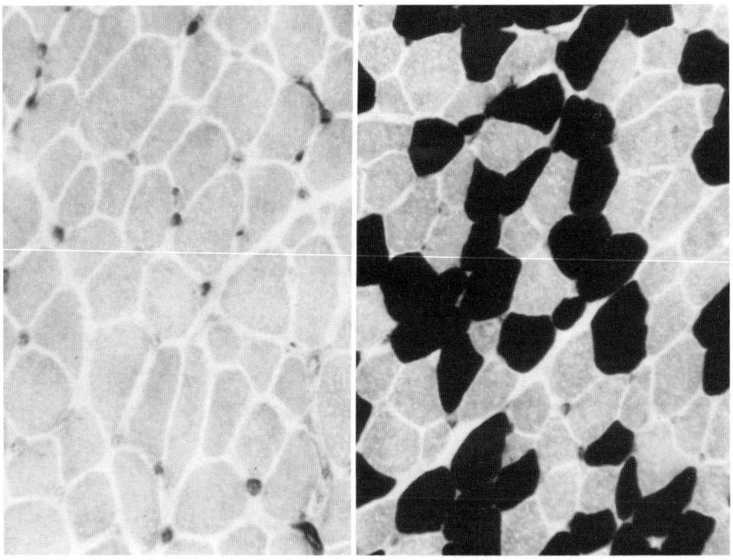

Fig. 5. Control (right) and paced (left) hemidiaphragm from 1 animal after continuous, low-frequency diaphragm stimulation. After alkaline (pH 10.1) preincubation, the ATPase reaction from a control hemidiaphragm shows a mixture of light (type I) and dark (type II) fibers in roughly equal proportions. The alkaline ATPase reaction from a paced hemidiaphragm shows a uniform population of light, low-activity type I fibers.

identified in paced specimens. Electron microscopic examination of control and paced hemidiaphragms showed no evidence of damage and preservation of normal ultrastructure with intact myofibrillary architecture and regular distribution of organelles [17]. No change in Z band width was seen but mitochondrial volume and capillary area increased.

Thus, this study suggests that continuous, low-frequency pacing of immature canine diaphragm alters both structure and function. To the extent that children using 12 or 24 h/day low-frequency pacing respond similarly, some predictions may be possible. The child's diaphragm should be converted from a mixed fiber-type muscle to one with nearly uniform characteristics. Oxidative enzymes should increase, and slow myosin isoforms should predominate. Diaphragmatic force and tidal volume generated should be maintained during low-frequency pacing but should decrease if tested at high stimulus frequencies.

Whether such changes in structure and function should be regarded as beneficial or deleterious depends on the function expected of the diaphragm. In both adults and children, low-frequency stimulation is adequate for maintenance of basal ventilation during sleep and quiet wakefulness [6, 12]. However, during periods of activity, infection or other increased demands on the diaphragm, loss of maximal force could be a significant disadvantage. It now seems possible that 24 h/day support of ventilation by diaphragm pacing is feasible for children. However, application of continuous diaphragm pacing should only be undertaken if it improves the quality of the child's life and then only by investigators experienced in the technique of pediatric diaphragm pacing.

Acknowledgement

The authors thank Michèle Fortin, Rosanna Barrafato, and John Gall for assistance preparing the manuscript.

References

1 Sarnoff SJ, Hardenbergh E, Whittenberger JL: Electrophrenic respiration. Am J Physiol 1948;155:1–9.
2 Glenn WWL, Phelps ML, Elefteriades JA, Dentz B, Hogan JF: Twenty years of experience in phrenic nerve stimulation to pace the diaphragm. PACE 1986;9:780–784.
3 Mellins RB, Balfour HH, Turino GM, Winters RW: Failure of automatic control of ventilation (Ondine's curse). Medicine 1970;49:487–504.
4 Hunt CE, Matalon SV, Thompson TR, Demuth S, Loew JM, Liu HM, Mastri A, Burke B: Central hypoventilation syndrome: Experience with bilateral phrenic nerve pacing in 3 neonates. Am Rev Respir Dis 1978;118:23–28.
5 Brouillette RT, Ilbawi MN, Hunt CE: Phrenic nerve pacing in infants and children: A review of experience and report on the usefulness of phrenic nerve stimulation studies. J Pediatr 1983;102:32–39.
6 Brouillette RT, Ilbawi MN, Klemka-Walden L, Hunt CE: Stimulus parameters for phrenic nerve pacing in infants and children. Pediatr Pulmonol 1988;4:33–38.
7 Weese-Mayer DE, Hunt CE, Brouillette RT, Silvestri JM: Diaphragm pacing in infants and children. J Pediatr 1992;120:1–8.
8 Ilbawi MN, Idriss FS, Hunt CE, Brouillette RT, DeLeon SY: Diaphragmatic pacing in infants: Techniques and results. Ann Thorac Surg 1985;40:323–329.
9 Marzocchi M, Brouillette RT, Weese-Mayer DE, Morrow AS, Conway LP: Comparison of transthoracic impedance/heart rate monitoring and pulse oximetry for patients using diaphragm pacemakers. Pediatr Pulmonol 1990;8:29–32.
10 Weese-Mayer DE, Morrow AS, Brouillette RT, Ilbawi MN, Hunt CE: Diaphragm pacing in infants and children: A life-table analysis of implanted components. Am Rev Respir Dis 1989;139:974–979.
11 Weese-Mayer DE, Brouillette RT, Naidich TP, McLone DG, Hunt CE: Magnetic resonance imaging and computerized tomography in central hyperventilation. Am Rev Respir Dis 1988;137:393–398.
12 Glenn WWL, Hogan JF, Loke JS, Ciesielski TE, Phelps ML, Rowedder R: Ventilatory support by pacing of the conditioned diaphragm in quadriplegia. N Engl J Med 1984;310:1150–1155.
13 Kim JH, Maneulids EE, Glenn WWL, Fukuda Y, Cole DG, Hogan JF: Light and electron microscopic studies of phrenic nerves after long-term electrical stimulation. J Neurosurg 1983;58:84–91.
14 Oda TW, Glenn WWL, Fukuda Y, Hogan JF, Gorfien J: Evaluation of electrical parameters for diaphragm pacing: An experimental study. J Surg Res 1981;30:142–153.
15 Ciesielski TE, Fukuda Y, Glenn WWL, Gorfien J, Jeffery K, Hogan JF: Response of the diaphragm muscle to electrical stimulation of the phrenic nerve. J Neurosurg 1983;58:92–100.
16 Marzocchi M, Brouillette RT, Klemka-Walden LM, Heller SL, Weese-Mayer DE, Brozanski BS, Caliendo J, Daood M, Ilbawi MN, Hunt CE: Effects of continuous low-frequency pacing on immature canine diaphragm. J Appl Physiol 1990;69:892–898.
17 Shah A, Sahgal V, Marzocchi M, Brouillette RT: Effects of diaphragmatic pacing in immature canine diaphragm. VII Int Conf Neuromusc Dis, Munich, 1990.

Biol Neonate 1994;65:272–280

Daniel Jordan
Nicolas Kopp

Lyon, France

Workshop

Definition and Criteria for Classification of Lesions Observed in Sudden Infant Death Syndrome for Further Research on the Central Nervous System: Proposal for a Consensus

Presentations

Beyond SIDS: A Pathology Profile of Infant Death

(J. Huber)

Since sudden infant death syndrome (SIDS) is defined as a diagnosis of exclusion, studies of it in isolation from other causes of sudden infant death have limited value. The group should consider the possibility that SIDS is a nonviable concept and that crib death be the focus of research.

It is recognized that a number of babies die (more or less) suddenly and unexpectedly. Even an extensive postmortem examination fails, in a number of cases, to reveal (major) pathological changes or recognized pathologically defined disease which can be regarded as a classifiable cause of death. However, establishing a classifiable cause of death does not necessarily mean that we have gained a clear insight into the precise mechanisms leading to death.

It is therefore important to organize the postmortem data of any deceased baby, irrespective of the mode of death (i.e. sudden or not) in such a way that insight is gained into:

1. Normality and the width of variation therefrom in regard to form, weight, measurements, histological and biochemical aspects of the body, the tissues and body fluids.
2. a) Disturbed body and organ growth.
   b) Disturbed development and differentiation of tissues.
   c) Congenital abnormalities, malformations.
   d) The role of exogenous factors.
   e) Familial hereditary and chromosomal background of a, b and c.
3. a) Pre- and perinatal insult.
   b) Complications of prematurity.
4. Lesions and abnormalities indicative of disturbed metabolism.
   a) Acute terminal events, the final common pathway.
   b) Of long duration, unknown or inborn error.
5. Immunological.
   a) Integrity.
   b) Reactivity-response.
   c) Atopy, allergy.
6. Infection.
   a) Bacterial.
   b) Viral.
   c) Tissue response to a and b.
7. Neoplasia.
8. Injury.
   a) Accidental.
   b) Nonaccidental.
   c) Iatrogenia.
9. Terminal responses, stresses.
10. Postmortem changes.

0006–3126/94/
0654–0272$5.00/0

It would furthermore be important to interpret and weigh the above data in a hierarchical and temporal manner as to their contribution to disease symptoms, disturbed physiological phenomena, and death. Duration and time of occurrence of lesions must be estimated.

Pathological, post- and antemortem studies in the human have the unique drawback that material is available only from dead or diseased tissue. The gathering of normal tissue is therefore of extreme importance but extrapolation from animal material is allowable with caution.

Particular emphasis must be laid, in view of the rapid development and differentiation in this age group, on gathering material from different age groups throughout gestation and the first year of life, both in normal controls and in subjects with well-defined pathological conditions.

With regard to the theme of the meeting, babies which suffered from hypoxia come to mind as well as babies known to have pre- and dysmaturity and perinatal insult.

It is proposed that the workshop considers and, in consensus, tries to find answers to the following:

(1) SIDS is a nonviable concept as a diagnosis or a syndrome, separate from and in exclusion of recognized classifiable disease entities. Study of so-called SIDS cases, in isolation, is a useless exercise.

(2) The broader term cot death (crib death, mort subite du nourrisson) covers a clinical phenomenon which shows a large overlap with known explained disease.

(3) For research purposes, a complete postmortem investigation of all infant deaths must include: (a) a full history from conception through pregnancy, parturition to postnatal development; (b) a family history; (c) a death scene investigation and estimation of time of death; (d) a full necropsy including gross and standard microscopical assessment of all organs; (e) bacteriological and virological survey; (f) biochemical assays; (g) freezing of designated (parts of) organs and body fluids; (h) fibroblast culture.

This applies also always when diagnosis of a clinical condition has been established prior to death.

(4) Sophisticated time-consuming and costly research methods should be applied exclusively to cases answering a description under 3.

(5) Normal control material should meet the same criteria as under 3.

(6) Can we define one final common pathway leading to death or is there more than one? If the latter, are there special pathways related to certain underlying pathological changes? What do we do with the concept of multifactorial origin of disease and death?

(7) How long does it take for various pathological changes to become established and be recognizable postmortem, i.e. disturbances in fluid distribution throughout the body, histological changes, changes in body fluids, electrolyte and pH changes, signs of hypoxia? Can we set time tables for the above?

(8) Which changes take place after death and over which tissue span? Can we set time limits for the postmortem interval after which certain investigations will become unreliable and which are these?

Clinical Experience and the Selection of Cerebral Structures to Be Investigated in SIDS Research

(A. Kahn)

Introduction

The physiology of the sudden infant and unexpected death of infants may be related to any of the following '3S': 'Sickness, Surroundings or Systems'. 'Sickness' refers to severe and fulminant disease processes, that may develop with few symptoms in previously healthy infants (such as septicemia, meningitis or myocarditis). 'Surrounding' includes all environmental factors exerting stressful challenges on the infant (such as overheating, sleep deprivation or sedative drugs). Finally, 'Systems' covers the various maturational processes developing during the early months of life, and potentially at risk of delay in maturation (such as cardiorespiratory or autonomic control mechanisms). Unexpected and unexplained deaths may occur because of any one of the three 'S' or of their combined effects. Only those cases for which no postmortem finding adequately explains the death are then defined as unexplained or 'SIDS' cases. The variability and paucity of signs that can be associated with these three 'S' may account for the difficulty to precisely assess the causal factor in many of the sudden infant deaths.

To contribute to the identification of cerebral structures to be investigated in SIDS research, we focus on the potential roles of obstructive sleep apneas (OSA) and of autonomic nervous system controls (ANS). Both could contribute to any of the above death processes.

Obstructive Sleep Apneas in Infants: Frequency and Mechanisms

Studies have shown that obstructive and mixed sleep apneas occur in less than 10% of healthy infants. Cinefluoroscopic and electromyographic findings indicate that during sleep apneas, the infant's tongue and hypopharyngeal soft tissues are approximately, obliterating the hypopharyngeal air space, with intermittent and almost complete obstruction of air flow.

The mechanisms of OSA are still debated. Some authors consider obstructive sleep apneas in children to be most frequently due to upper airway anatomic abnormalities, such as bone malformations, soft tissue infiltration, and/or neurologic lesions impairing muscle contractions. In premature and young infants, stimulation of pressure-sensitive and chemosensitive receptors may also induce apneas. Environmental factors, such as body position, neck flexion, sleep deprivation or the use of sedatives could all contribute. Neurologic abnormalities associated with OSA include seizure, increased intracranial pressure, spinal cord compressions, palsy of the cranial nerves or poliomyelitis.

Possible Relation between OSA and SIDS

OSA have been associated with SIDS. Family members of SIDS victims may suffer from obstructive apneas, due to the presence of small airways, or a loss of tonic genioglossus activity during sleep. Infants have been reported to die some days after the accidental recording of repeated OSA. Prospective polygraphic studies have shown that future SIDS victims have more frequent and longer obstructive apneas during sleep than control infants. Postmortem findings in some SIDS victims reveal thickening of the basement membrane of the vocal cords, possibly related to repeated global closure. Rabbits dying from imposed airway obstruction have postmortem findings of SIDS, including pulmonary edema and pleural petechiae.

The Role of the Autonomic Nervous Controls in the Development of OSA

The autonomic nervous system could play a role in the development of OSA. OSA was reported in children suffering from various congenital or acquired autonomic nervous system disorders, such as familial dysautonomia, or breath-holding spells. Atropine has occasionally been reported to prevent OSA.

The Role of the ANS in the Development of SIDS

During sleep, SIDS victims were reported to exhibit symptoms that could be related to ANS dysfunctions. Tachycardia, bradycardia, decreased heart rate variability, prolonged Q-Tc index, profuse sweating, or changes in skin color were reported. During feeding, some future SIDS victims display poor coordination of swallowing and breathing.

Postmortem Findings Compatible with a Role for the ANS in SIDS

Both the sympathetic and the vagal components of the ANS have been implicated in the development of SIDS. Autopsies on infants that died of SIDS have shown abnormalities in the myelinization of fine fibers in the vagus nerve, abnormal proliferation of astrocytic fibers in the central nervous system, abnormal reticular formations from the brain stem, or abnormal persistence of reticular, dendritic endings. These anatomical features could be related to the neurological, respiratory or cardiac disorders seen in some victims of SIDS.

Conclusions

The contributing role of the ANS and of the OSA in some cases of SIDS may not be excluded, but need further evaluation. Postmortem and animal studies of the structures and pathways responsible for the control of the autonomic system, and of upper airway patency could bring further insight into some of the potential mechanisms of SIDS.

Pathological Data in Sudden Infant Death Autopsies

(C. Rambaud)

The sudden unexpected death (SUD, cot death) is a natural death which occurs suddenly or very quickly in an infant under 1 year of age, apparently in good health. In 1969, Beckwith defined the sudden infant death syndrome (SIDS) as a death which remains unexplained after complete postmortem investigations including autopsy. This definition was reviewed in Sydney (SIDS International Meeting, February 1992), with recommendations for its administrative and medical use.

The main problem comes from this definition and concerns what is accepted as a cause of death. This induces a large variation between 20 and 80% in nonexplained death according to different teams. Most of them mix sudden unexpected death and unexplained death.

Whatever the percentage of death causes kept in SUD, the objective epidemiological and pathological published data are the same. The common points of these deaths are age (85% are under 4 months of life), death circumstances (in the crib), and superposition with seasonal infection curves. Inflammatory lesions, especially in the lungs, are very frequent. Necker-Enfants Malades Hospital is 1 of the 2 SUD Paris area reference centers since 1986. Investigations of the dead infants are always made with the same pluridisciplinary protocol [1]. After the autopsy, results are graded into 4 groups:

Group A when we found a cause of death (significant lesions are made by their feature or their severity); group B when there are significant lesions but not enough to explain the death; group C for minor lesions, and group D when nothing is found. We find a cause for the death in almost 80% of the cases.

The main pathological group A lesions are pulmonary and cardiac.

The pulmonary lesions form the major part. The lungs are fixed in a formaldehyde solution after having been slashed, without any further manipulation. The histological study is performed on 7 slides (one of each lobe and one of each hilum). We consider the following lesions to be a cause of death when they are present on all slides:

(a) No more alveolar air, which can be the consequence either of major inflammatory lesions (alveolar, interstitial or combined inflammation), either by diffuse alveolar edema or hemorrhage. In case of interstitial inflammatory lesions, the aeration loss can only come from increased alveolar wall thickness. (b) Bronchiolitis, even isolated, if it is important and diffuse. (c) Alimentary material aspiration when it is found in most of the bronchi and bronchioli, invading alveolar spaces, associated with vital reaction, and this even in case of prolonged resuscitation operations so long as no cardiac activity has been reestablished. (d) Pulmonary embolism in a large arterial branch, or numerous distal embolisms.

In our series (167 SUD aged from 1 month to 1 year, between 1986 and 1991), the pulmonary pathology has been considered as responsible for the death in 46% of the cases. There were 63 cases with no more aeration (32 heavy pneumonitis, interstitial, alveolar or combined); 7 major pulmonary hemorrhage; 24 massive pulmonary edema – 19 of which were the consequence of a cardiac or neurological pathology discovered at autopsy – 11 alimentary material aspirations, 2 isolated bronchiolitis, and 1 idiopathic pulmonary embolism. Only 7 lungs were normal. The histological inflammatory lesions have been connected with a simultaneous infectious disease. In the same period, a pathogenic agent has been identified in one-third of the cases, with an equal viral and bacterial distribution.

The cardiac lesions, inflammatory and noninflammatory, also by themselves explain a lot of deaths.

Myocarditis is frequent (almost 17% in our series). Diagnosis is made according to the Dallas criteria, which associates an inflammatory infiltrate to a cellular necrosis (or its equivalents). Numerous samples are needed because of the focal and slightly inflammatory nature of the infiltrate. Indeed, as in endomyocardial biopsies, it can be responsible for false-negative diagnosis if the sampling is not sufficient. We usually take 7 samples, with a particular focus to the core septal area, which is an inflammatory infiltrate's preferential location. The noninflammatory cardiac lesions are less frequent (aroud 3.5% in our series) and consist of cardiomyopathies, tumors more often in the septal zone, myocardial diffuse fibrosis, unknown congenital cardiopathies, myocardial focal hemorrhage and necrosis.

The other autopsy lesions seen in the A group are heterogeneous. In our series, among macroscopical lesions, there are diffuse digestive hemorrhages in the whole small bowel, one hemorrhage in the central nervous system, 2 massive dehydrations, rickets with major craniotabes. Among histological lesions, there are several meningitis (meningitis diagnosis is made only on polynuclear inflammation), exceptional encephalitis, some myopathies, rare metabolic disorders, and one lymphohistiocytosis.

The anatomobiological and microbiological meeting is essential, bringing clinical radiological and/or microbiological elements. These confirm the infants' pathological data which were classified into group A, or allow to explain the death when the data alone were not sufficient to do it (groups B, C and D). In particular, this is the case for septicemia or meningitis which could induce only a few histological lesions, or in the case of infants dying of hyperthermia or being buried beneath the covers.

To find a cause of death does not inevitably mean having found the cause of the death. It is currently admitted by all authors that these deaths are of multifactorial origin. At the moment, the unexplained SUD remains unexplained only within the actual state of the investigation. Indeed, the concept of SIDS or unexplained infant death has to be reviewed. Because of that, it is not evident that infants found dead in their cots could be divided into 2 opposite groups: a control group made up of the explained or partially explained death and a group of the fully unexplained deaths. The aim is to identify the physiological factor(s) which made the infant so sensitive to infections, without the typical signs of alarm. The search for central nervous system abnormalities, morphological and especially biochemical, is made most difficult by the changes due to death and by the postmortem hypoxia of the infants dying from severe respiratory infections.

Reference

1 Rambaud C, Imbert MC: Protocole d'autopsie d'une mort subite du nourrisson. Ann Pathol 1993;13:131–134.

A Perspective on Neuropathologic Findings in Victims of the Sudden Infant Death Syndrome (SIDS): The Triple-Risk Model

(J.J. Filiano)

SIDS is characterized by the sudden infant death of an apparently healthy infant during a sleep period which occurs in the first few months of postnatal life. The broad hypothesis that SIDS is due to a central or peripheral abnormality in cardiopulmonary control mechanisms has generated many neuropathologic studies which we recently reviewed. The major central nervous system (CNS) findings include subtle brain stem gliosis (scarring), increased brain stem dendritic spine density, decreased levels of neurotransmitters or their biosynthetic enzymes within and above brain stem regions, increased number of ALZ-50 immunostained neurons in the hippocampus, hypoplasia of the arcuate nucleus, periventricular leukomalacia, cerebral white matter gliosis, subtle hypomyelination, megaloencephaly, cerebral edema, and decreased cerebrospinal fluid melatonin. While it is not clear how (or if) these findings relate to one another or to the pathogenesis of sudden death, taken together they support the concept that all SIDS victims are not entirely 'normal', but rather may possess underlying vulnerabilities which put them at risk for sudden death. The concept of a vulnerable infant forms a key link in a triple-risk model suggested by us for the pathogenesis of SIDS. This model proposes that SIDS results from the intersection of three overlapping factors:

(1) a vulnerable infant; (2) a critical developmental period, and (3) an exogenous stressor(s).

According to this model, an infant will die of SIDS only if he/she possesses all three factors. The temporal association of sudden death with a sleep period further suggests that the infant's vulnerability lies in homeostatic control during sleep or in the transition between sleep and waking. The idea of a critical developmental period is based on epidemiologic data indicating a consistent age distribution for SIDS, with a peak at 2–4 months. During this period, major changes occur in virtually all physiological systems, including autonomic control, ventilation and state organization, as infants attain adaptative mechanisms enabling them to maintain homeostasis in the face of extrauterine stresses. Potential stressors which have been linked to SIDS include minor respiratory or gastrointestinal illnesses, fever, hyperthermia induced by over-blanketing, and prone sleeping position. The triple-risk model proposes that the infant's vulnerability lies latent until he/she enters the critical developmental period and is subject to an exogenous stressor which overwhelms the already compromised homeostatic system. According to this model, heterogenous disorders may make the infant vulnerable to sudden death during the critical period. Given this possibility, it is not unexpected that the same neuropathologic findings are not present in all SIDS victims, nor represent a single entity which 'explains' all SIDS deaths. The neuropathologic findings in individual cases may reflect the primary site and/or mechanism of injury in a homeostatic control system, or be secondary to an underlying defect, for example in energy metabolism, which results both in sudden death and brain abnormalities. Neuropathologic findings, however subtle, should be vigorously pursued, because they may provide the clues towards deciphering the potentially diverse vulnerabilities in affected infants (supported by the National Sudden Infant Death Syndrome Alliance, Hearst Foundation and National Institute of Child Health and Human Development).

Sudden Infant Death Syndrome Research in the US: Attempts at Classification Criteria

(M. Willinger)

The National Institute of Child Health and Human Development (NICHD) of the National Institutes of Health has primary Federal responsibility for research on the sudden infant death syndrome. Program objectives are to understand the causes and underlying mechanisms of the syndrome; to identify infants at risks for becoming victims; to clarify the relationship between high-risk pregnancy, high-risk infancy and SIDS; to explore preventive approaches and ultimately to prevent sudden infant deaths. In 1988, the United States Senate requested 'that NICHD prepare and submit a report detailing a 5-year SIDS research plan ...'. NICHD is currently implementing the third year of the plan submitted to Congress. It outlines activities in the fields of epidemiology, neonatology, cardiorespiratory and sleep research, neuroscience, infectious diseases and immunology, pathology and metabolic diseases.

In 1989, NICHD convened a workshop to determine whether progress has been sufficient to revise current criteria for SIDS diagnosis, particularly for those cases which serve as a base for research on SIDS. A revised definition of SIDS was published this year in *Pediatric Pathology* [1991;11:677–684], as follows: 'The sudden death of an infant under one year of age which remains unexplained after performance of a complete postmortem investigation, including an autopsy, examination of the death scene, and review of the case history.'

The efforts of the NICHD to standardize diagnosis and tissue collection encompass the following.

(1) A SIDS histopathology atlas has been generated from microscopic and quantitative analysis of histologic specimens from the NICHD collaborative SIDS epidemiologic study. A collection of formalin-fixed tissues from the study is available for research.

(2) A Brain and Tissue Bank for Developmental Disorders has been established at the University of Maryland to collect and store specimens from 'unaffected' fetuses, infants and children and those with neurodevelopmental disorders, including SIDS victims. A standard database and neuropathology protocol has been developed. The repositories will distribute tissue to qualified investigators to conduct investigations that will lead to improved understanding of the causes of SIDS and the abnormalities of SIDS victims.

(3) A multicenter study of high-risk infants is underway to determine whether home apnea monitors employing event recordings are effective in identifying clinically relevant episodes and to develop a profile of a physiologic high-risk infant. A standard autopsy and death scene protocol will be used.

(4) A case control study of all sudden infant deaths among native Americans in the Aberdeen area of the Indian Health Service is being initiated to accurately identify the causes of infant death; obtain information about medical, environmental and social factors that may be responsible for the high rate of infant death, and improve public health support for families experiencing an infant death. A standard death scene investigation and autopsy protocol will be used and an in-depth neuropathologic analysis will be conducted on every case.

(5) The interagency Panel on SIDS will review and establish updated standard death scence and autopsy protocols for sudden infant deaths for the nation at the request of the United States Senate.

(6) The International Working Groups of the Global Strategy Task Force on SIDS, established in 1992, serve as vehicles for future cooperative efforts. The activities of the Pathology International Working Group encompass the development of a proposal for an international definition of SIDS; the development of standardized autopsy and event scene investigation protocols; the development of a proposal for an international tissue exchange, and an international computerized database with elements of the postmortem investigations of infant deaths.

In my view, SIDS cases should be classified quite strictly as outlined in *Pediatric Pathology*. Therefore, cases failing to meet the standards of this definition, including those without a postmortem investigation, should not be diagnosed as SIDS. Cases that are autopsied and carefully investigated, but which remain unresolved may be designated as 'undetermined', 'unexplained' or the like. For example, some cases of pneumonia which might be considered as probable or possible SIDS, should be diagnosed as 'in question, possible pneumonia'. However, research studies should be broadened to include infant deaths from as many diagnoses as possible, including those in question, to get a sense of the prevalence of a particular lesion. In addition, cases should be matched for gestational age.

Workshop Discussion: Consensus

(1) Same approach for all cases from birth to 1 year old (postconceptional age) + fetuses (20–40 weeks old), including specific diseases like Ondine's curse, Pierre Robin, Down's syndrome, familial dysautonomia, etc.

(2) Research would direct the cases you investigated and selected for that particular aim.

(3) Common basic autopsy protocol. Participants: Prof. Huber, only a summary of the final synthesis done by Prof. Huber will be given here. Detailed forms (23 pages) will be available on request.

Summary of postmortem protocol (infants 0–365 days)
I. Administrative-nominative data All further pages to be identified only by local number and international registry
II. Preliminary information a) Short history b) First examination by doctors who pronounce death c) First laboratory workup
III. Autopsy protocol Routine – gross and macroscopic Special studies a) Toxicology b) Bacteriology c) Virology d) Chemistry e) Fibroblast culture f) Tissues/materials frozen or fixed for storage
IV. Detailed history
V. Summary and final conclusions Final diagnoses
VI. Support of the family Recommendations

(4) Postmortem delay and use of the brain. Participants: Prof. Oehmichen, synthesis of participants' requirements.

	Immuno-histo-chemistry	Auto-radiographic receptors	In situ hybridi-zation	Bio-chemical studies
Consensus on postmortem delay, h	≤12	≤24	≤12	≤12

Postmortem delay is defined as the time (in h) between the time of death (mean time between last seen alive and discovered death) and the time the tissue sample is fixed or kept frozen at –80 °C. Brain: weigh fresh.

(5) Histology (formalin-fixed brain).

Spinal cord	Cervical enlargment (C4 included)

Brain stem	Medulla
	  Mid olive
	  Obex
	Pons includes
	  Level of superior cerebellar peduncle
	Mesencephalon
	  Decussatio superior cerebellar peduncle
	  Level of red nucleus

Cerebellum	At 45° with dendate

Cerebral hemispheres	Left side
	  Frontal pole
	  Head caudate (+ corpus callosum lateral ventricle)
	  Thalamus (+ corpus mammillare + lenticular)
	  Hippocampus: mid portion
	  Calcarine fissures
	Right side
	  Save for banking system

Anatomical sampling: according to the atlas of R. Nieuwenhuys, 'The Human Central Nervous System: A Synopsis and Atlas', 3rd revised edition, Springer Verlag.

(6) Pineal (fixed).
(7) Pituitary (frozen at −80 °C).

Dr. Jordan's Recommendations

When the brain has been removed (and rapidly weighed in the fresh state), one might observe while viewing the base of the skull, the pituitary stalk emerging from the diaphragma sellae. In order to remove the pituitary gland, paying attention to preserve its integrity, one might proceed as follows: cut the diaphragma sellae with a sharp knife around its junction with the base of skull (be careful not to damage the pituitary gland underneath) and remore it. The pituitary gland is then visible with the pituitary stalk still in place. At that point carefully take off the pituitary gland with Taylor forceps (straight serated tips) by gently separating it from the sellae starting at the tuberculum down to the walls to the bottom of the sellae, gently cutting off adherences with a sharp knife (one might use iris spatulae to help) to the anterior, posterior and lateral walls of the sellae. The removed pituitary gland is then layed in an anatomical position (pituitary stalk up) on a microscope slide and store at −80 °C inside a sealed plastic flask to protect it against lyophilisation.

(8) Miscellaneous
- Adrenals (frozen, left side; fixed, right side).
- Phrenic nerve (frozen, fixed).
- Sympathetic of heart: left ventricle (frozen); right atrium including the sinusoidal nodose (frozen).
- Septum of heart: 1/3 superior part – anterior part (fixed); posterior part (frozen).
- Fluids: CSF – 3 samples of 500 µl + EDTA 10 m*M* (final concentration); 3 samples of 200 µl per autopsy, suboccipital recommended. Serum – 3 samples of 500 µl + EDTA 10 m*M* (final concentration); 3 samples of 200 µl intracardiac puncture by right laterosternal puncture.
- Choroid plexus: lateral ventricle (frozen, fixed).
- Thymus (frozen).

(9) Brain stem (frozen; 12 h < pmd < 24 h; fixed: pmd < 12 h, pmd = postmortem delay).

(10) Brain hemispheric sections
- Two hemispheric sections (frozen, banking system; fixed, diagnostic).
- Hippocampus (frozen, left side: 1 cm, mid-portion; fixed, right side).
- Occipital cortex (frozen, fixed).
- Cerebellum after removing the brain stem (frozen, fixed).

(11) Autoradiography studies (frozen – 80 °C).
Brain stem + cervical spinal cord – C4 (included).

(12) DNA measurement when possible.

(13) Banking system.

Each participant or center is required to send detailed information about their banking activities (material, storage, database) to Prof. T.O. Rognum, who is in charge of banking system organisation for the Pathology International Working Group of the SIDS Global Strategy Task Force. Prof. Rognum is in the process of developing a computerized network of existing pediatric tissue banks, which include banks focusing on the nervous system. Potential users should contact him for information regarding available tissues.

The presently existing banking in Oslo concerns both SIDS and controls material fixed or frozen at −80 °C. As far as database is concerned, information about cases are recorded on database: DATABASE, the equipment used in IBM compatible.

(14) Sample storage (frozen (−80 °C): 2 years; fixed: 5 years, paraformaldehyde 4%, 0.1 *M*, pH 7.4, if impossible, formaldehyde).

Ebook Set up and Use Instructions

Use of the ebook is subject to the single user licence at the back of this book.

Electronic access to your price book is now provided as an ebook on the VitalSource® Bookshelf platform. You can access it online or offline on your PC/Mac, smartphone or tablet. You can browse and search the content across all the books you've got, make notes and highlights and share these notes with other users.

Setting up

1. Create a VitalSource Bookshelf account at https://online.vitalsource.com/user/new (or log into your existing account if you already have one).

2. Retrieve the code by scratching off the security-protected label inside the front cover of this book. Log in to Bookshelf and click the **Redeem Codes link in the Tools** menu at the top right of the screen. Enter the code in the **Redeem code** box and press **Redeem**. Once the code has been redeemed your Spon's Price Book will download and appear in your **library**. N.B. the code in the scratch-off panel can only be used once.

When you have created a Bookshelf account and redeemed the code you will be able to access the ebook online or offline on your smartphone, tablet or PC/Mac. Your notes and highlights will automatically stay in sync no matter where you make them.

Use ONLINE

1. Log in to your Bookshelf account at https://online.vitalsource.com).
2. Double-click on the title in your **library** to open the ebook.

Use OFFLINE

Download BookShelf to your PC, Mac, iOS device, Android device or Kindle Fire, and log in to your Bookshelf account to access your ebook, as follows:

On your PC/Mac
Go to https://support.vitalsource.com/hc/en-us/categories/360001056774-Bookshelf#360002383594 and follow the instructions to download the free VitalSource Bookshelf app to your PC or Mac. Double-click the VitalSource Bookshelf icon that appears on your desktop and log into your Bookshelf account. Select **All Titles** from the menu on the left – you should see your price book on your Bookshelf. If your Price Book does not appear, select **Update Booklist** from the **Account** menu. Double-click the price book to open it.

On your iPhone/iPod Touch/iPad
Download the free VitalSource Bookshelf App available via the iTunes App Store. Open the Bookshelf app and log into your Bookshelf account. Select **All Titles** – you should see your price book on your Bookshelf. Select the price book to open it. You can find more information at https://support.vitalsource.com/hc/en-us/articles/360014105113-iOS

On your Android™ smartphone or tablet
Download the free VitalSource Bookshelf App available via Google Play. Open the Bookshelf app and log into your Bookshelf account. You should see your price book on your Bookshelf. Select the price book to open it. You can find more information at https://support.vitalsource.com/hc/en-us/articles/360014007294-Android

On your Kindle Fire
Download the free VitalSource Bookshelf App from Amazon. Open the Bookshelf app and log into your Bookshelf account. Select All Titles – you should see your price book on your Bookshelf. Select the price book to open it. You can find more information at https://support.vitalsource.com/hc/en-us/articles/360014107953-Kindle-Fire

Support

If you have any questions about downloading Bookshelf, creating your account, or accessing and using your ebook edition, please visit https://support.vitalsource.com/

For questions or comments on content, please contact us on sponsonline@tandf.co.uk

---